The Complete Guide to

NAVY
SEAL
FITNESS

The Complete Guide to

NAVY SEAL FITNESS

LT. Stewart Smith, USN (SEAL)

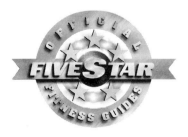

Five Star Publishing
An Independent Imprint of Hatherleigh Press

Five Star Publishing
1114 First Avenue, Suite 500
New York, NY 10021
1-800-906-1234
www.getfitnow.com

The use of the words Navy SEALs does not imply nor infer an endorsement, either explicit or implicit, by the United States Navy or the Navy SEALs.

Before beginning any strenuous exercise program consult your physician. The author and publisher of this book and workout disclaim any liability, personal or professional, resulting from the misapplication of any of the training procedures described in this publication.

A portion of the proceeds from the sale of each book will be donated to the Make-A-Wish Foundation.

All Five Star Publishing titles are available for bulk purchase, special promotions, and premiums. For more information, please contact the manager of our Special Sales Department at 1-800-906-1234.

Library of Congress Cataloging-in-Publication Data

Smith, Stewart. 1969–
    The complete guide to Navy SEAL fitness / Stewart Smith.
        p.   cm.
    ISBN 1-57826-014-0 (alk. paper)
    1. United States. Navy. SEALs. 2. Exercise. 3. Physical
    fitness.   I. Title.
    GV481.S644   1998
    613.7—dc21   97-46559
                                                                                       CIP

Cover design by Gary Szczecina
Text design and composition by John Reinhardt Book Design
Photographed by Peter Field Peck with Canon® cameras
and lenses on Fuji® print and slide film

Printed on acid-free paper
10 9 8 7 6 5 4 3 2

DEDICATION

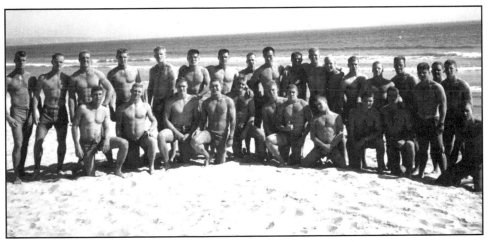

BUD/S Class 182—"Wet and Sandy"

The Complete Guide to Navy SEAL Fitness is dedicated to those
men who have chosen a profession most men would not dare . . .

To those men who do every day what most men
would not dream of doing . . .

To those men who understand what it means to
"never leave your swim buddy" . . .

And to those who have given their lives in the service of their country.

HOOYAH to the US Navy Frogmen past and present!

ACKNOWLEDGMENTS

How do I begin to say thank you to the many people who have helped me in the past, who have shown me the right path to follow in life? I could fill several pages with names of family members, friends, SEALs, and other Naval Officers and Enlisted to whom I am grateful.

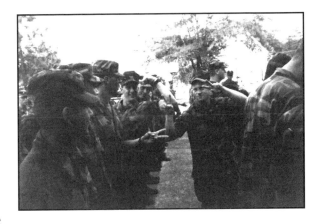

First and foremost—my family has been absolutely supportive in all the endeavors I have chosen. Thank you Mom, Dad, and Liz for always believing in me when the chances were slim that I would succeed. You gave me the strength to TRY, which has led to my SUCCESS. My wife Denise, who has been with me since I was a Midshipman, has given me the will and the desire to strive for excellence every day. Denise and my new child have given me the energy and motivation to prepare for the future by working hard today.

My best friend from my hometown of Live Oak, FL—Keith Bonds has and always will be a friend, no matter how long I am away. Through his steadfast friendship and comic relief, I have learned to enjoy life by relaxing and watching the Suwannee River slowly roll past. My best friend in the TEAMS, LT. Alden Mills, and I have been together since we met on restriction our sophomore year at USNA. Through BUD/S, Advanced Training, SDV Team TWO Task Unit Alpha, and who knows what else, he has always been there for me no matter what.

The enlisted men of the SEAL Teams have made a huge impact on my life. Their dedication to duty and their loyalty to their shipmates has made an unforgettable mark on my work ethic and enjoyment of missions accomplished. Thanks for your energy! I wish I could list all of you, but I risk forgetting one of the many of you who has been my swim buddy, point man, or a good friend. You know who you are. The many senior officers, who lead by example, have made an impression that will last a lifetime. To my "Sea-Daddy" CDR Tom Joyce—I have learned so much from your leadership and your example of what a Navy family should be.

I thank God for giving me the ability to accomplish what I have. With the strength God has given me, I can only hope to help others achieve their personal goals. That is why I wrote this book—to receive the rewarding feeling of helping another reach their goals.

— STEWART SMITH
December, 1997

CONTENTS

Preface   **11**

Introduction   **15**
　Preparing for SEAL Training   16
　About BUD/S   18
　Mental Preparation   21

Stretching   **25**

Physical Training   **51**
　Upper Body Exercises   52
　Lower Body Exercises   60
　Abdominal Exercises   66

Pull-ups and Dips   **77**

Running at BUD/S   **87**

Swimming at BUD/S   **91**

Rope Climbing: Just for Fun   **99**

The 12 Weeks to BUD/S Workout   **103**

If You Are a Beginner . . .   **137**

About the Author   **151**

PREFACE

The **Complete Guide to Navy SEAL Fitness** is a progressive, 12-week workout designed for individuals who are interested in becoming Navy SEALs or for people who like an extremely challenging workout. It is filled with pictures of stretches and exercises, running and swimming techniques, and a chapter on what to expect during SEAL training, as well as weekly workout charts that specifically guide you through some of the toughest workouts known. The unique concept of this workout regimen is that it requires no weight room equipment. You do not need to buy any equipment! All you need is a place to run, swim, and perform pull-ups and dips. Most school playgrounds or local parks have the necessary equipment.

This is the same workout that I perform with the midshipmen at the US Naval Academy who attend Basic Underwater Demolition/ SEAL Training (BUD/S) after graduation. Over thirty U.S. Naval Academy graduates have used this workout and all have had 100% completion records. This is a remarkable accomplishment, particularly when over 75% of BUD/S students traditionally quit.

Every year there are thousands of American teenagers who want to become Navy SEALs. There are also millions of Americans who want a challenging workout that does not require a membership fee. This workout not only physically challenges and prepares you for the toughest military training in the world, but also mentally prepares you by building your confidence and strength.

The Complete Guide to Navy SEAL Fitness also prepares you to ace the SEAL Physical Fitness Test (PFT) by measuring your fitness level every month as you take a practice SEAL PFT.

The Complete Guide to Navy SEAL Fitness starts at an intermediate level of fitness. In each of the first ten weeks, the exercise repetitions increase. The final two weeks taper off in order to prevent burnout from such high levels of intense training. I have also included a four-week "Pre-Training Phase" to help beginners build the strength and endurance that will be needed for the 12-week SEAL workout.

Chapters on how to run in the sand and swim with fins take this workout a step further. An elementary lesson on the sidestroke, the most common swim stroke at BUD/S, is vital if you are to successfully complete the 12-week training program. An instructional video on how to better your swim times for the SEAL PFT and how to swim with fins utilizing the uncommon sidestroke is also available.

If you follow and finish this 12-week workout, you will most likely find yourself in the best physical shape of your life. Finishing won't be easy, but with determination, you will make it. And wait until you see the results. Good luck!

INJURY DISCLAIMER

Before beginning any strenuous exercise program consult your physician. The author and
publisher of **The Complete Guide to Navy
SEAL Fitness** workout disclaim any liability, personal or professional, resulting
from the misapplication of any of the
training procedures described in this
publication. Take your health and fitness seriously!

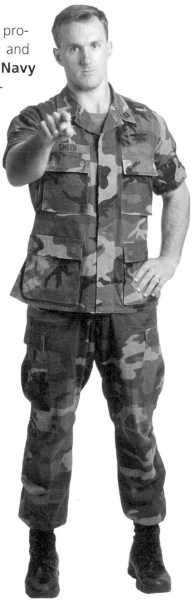

INTRODUCTION

This Workout *Will* Prepare You For SEAL Training OR Anything Else!

Any well-conditioned person can do these workouts. There are over 70 different combinations of workouts included in this book, with pictures of stretches, exercises, running, and swimming. Over 150 pictures teach you every exercise as well as the proper techniques for running, swimming, and training with the world's fittest individuals—The US Navy SEALs!

You might ask, how does this workout prepare me for anything else? Believe it or not, if you can successfully complete this 12-week workout challenge, you will be physically prepared for ANY other military training. From Basic training—Army, Navy, Air Force, Marine Corps—to advanced military training like BUD/S, this workout will physically prepare you to do them all! Even if you have no desire to be in the military, but enjoy working out every day, **The Complete Guide to Navy SEAL Fitness** will definitely get you into top physical condition.

More importantly, the unbelievable amount of confidence you will gain in your abilities will change your life. Never before have you been able to do 750 pushups in one workout or complete the exhausting four-mile run–one-mile swim–three-mile run in an hour and a half, but with this progressive step-by-step exercise program you will be conquering what you thought was impossible. You have no idea how this will affect your personal and professional life! You will gain confidence in your abilities that people will notice. Your boss, friends, and co-workers will see a lean, fit, self-assured person who has the attitude that anything can be accomplished. You will feel like you have never felt before in your life. You will have the energy to work all day, come home, play with the kids, or do whatever else needs to be done.

Let's face it. First impressions are lasting impressions. When you walk into a room full of people, the first thing they notice is your appearance—your height, weight, and physique. When you finish this workout, your physical appearance will command respect immediately; then, as you start mingling and talking to people, your words and actions will exude confidence. This is the biggest advantage you can have over your peers—confidence. Does this workout automatically give you confidence? NO! But it will help you build your confidence, just as it helps you build your strength and stamina.

Preparing for SEAL Training (BUD/S)

The primary goal of this workout program is to prepare and teach individuals about the challenges they will face at Basic Underwater Demolition/SEAL training (BUD/S). The secondary goal is to provide men and women with a progressively difficult 12-week workout that will challenge them everyday. If you are a tri-athlete or a hardcore workout animal, you will enjoy this workout. THIS IS NOT A WORKOUT FOR BEGINNERS! You must be in shape long before you attempt this program. These workouts focus on running, swimming, and Physical Training (PT). PT, also known as calisthenics, is comprised of high-repetition, muscle- and stamina-building exercises that will make you leaner and more muscular than you have ever dreamed.

To achieve the primary goal of this workout, you have to be prepared to take the SEAL "Entrance Exam," also known as the SEAL Physical Fitness Test, or PFT. It consists of the following:

500 yard swim using the side or breaststroke	(10 minute rest)
Maximum number of Pushups in 2 minutes	(2 minute rest)
Maximum number of Situps in 2 minutes	(2 minute rest)
Maximum number of Pull-ups	(10 minute rest)
1.5 mile run in boots and pants	

This alone is a tough workout! Every fourth week during the 12-week workout, you will take the SEAL PFT in order to check your progress. You may see that your scores do not change the third and fourth time you take the PFT. This is because you are in the toughest weeks of the workout and are actually burned out (if you are doing all the exercises). But do not fear, because during weeks 10–12, a three-week tapering of intensity takes place and you will rebuild your strength and speed. After the twelfth week, start over at Week One and take the SEAL PFT. After your three-week taper, you will see a huge increase in your numbers and a decrease in your times.

The three-week taper is in the workout in order to prevent over-training. If you are supplementing this workout with heavy weight-lifting workouts, longer swims, and runs during the "easy" weeks, you will NOT see the huge gains that a well-rested athlete will experience.

Below are the minimum times needed to pass the SEAL PFT. As you can see, these scores are not that tough to achieve. However, a person who obtains just the minimum scores will not have a chance to get into BUD/S, due to the enormous competition of highly qualified applicants. The competitive scores are the above average scores that I have seen from men who get accepted into BUD/S. The best scores I have seen are from those incredible athletes you will compete with and work with when you are at BUD/S.

	Minimum Scores	Competitive Range	Best Scores I've Seen
Swim (min.)	12:30	7:00–8:30	5:45 sidestroke
Pushups	42	100–120	150
Situps	50	100–120	135
Pull-ups	8	20–30	42
1.5 Mile (min.)	11:30	8:30–10:00	7:45

Though there are no maximum scores for this "Entrance Exam," it is highly recommended that you give your best effort in all areas, in order to be competitive for this highly sought-after course of instruction.

Your number of pull-ups, pushups, and situps will increase after the 12-week workout. Your 1.5-mile-run time will decrease as you train to get your legs and lungs stronger than they have ever been. Your time for the 500-yard sidestroke or breaststroke swim will also decrease due to the large amount of swimming you will do. Detailed pictures and descriptions of the swimming strokes you will use at BUD/S will help you to perfect your technique.

About BUD/S

Basic Underwater Demolition/SEAL (BUD/S) training is one of the most physically demanding military programs in the world. BUD/S lasts for twenty-six weeks, with each week getting harder and harder. No one graduates from BUD/S without being challenged in some way. It is impossible to meet all the different demands of BUD/S without mentally pushing yourself to succeed. Graduating from BUD/S is possible (thousands have been successful), but ask any SEAL and they will tell you that something personally challenged them to dig deep within and push themselves to succeed. This is why BUD/S is called the "toughest military training in the world."

BUD/S is divided into three phases. Descriptions of each phase are below:

First Phase (Basic Conditioning)

First Phase lasts for nine weeks. The first four weeks test you in the areas of soft-sand running in boots, swimming with fins in the ocean, and doing more pull-ups, pushups, and flutter kicks than you have ever imagined doing. On the average, a member of your class will quit each day during the first four weeks. The fifth week is known as "Hell Week." During this week, BUD/S students endure 120 hours of continuous training, with minimal sleep (a total 3–4 hours—for the entire week). Also known as "Motivational Week," this week is designed to be the ultimate test of the student's physical and mental desire to become a SEAL. Typically, fifty percent of your class will quit or be medically discharged by the time Hell Week is over.

Why do Hell Week?

The experience of Hell Week is what SEALs draw from when situations are cold, dark, and miserable. It proves to all SEALs that the human body can do ten times the amount of work and endure ten times the amount of pain and discomfort than the average human thinks possible. SEALs learn how to remain calm and react properly in hostile situations; how to persevere in the face of adversity; and most importantly, they learn the value of teamwork. The last three weeks of First Phase are spent learning hydrographic reconnaissance and recuperating a little from your 120-hour personal test. Rarely do men quit after Hell Week.

Second Phase (Diving)

Diving Phase lasts for seven weeks. During this period, physical training continues and the workouts get harder. Students have to run their four-mile runs a minute faster, swim their two-mile swims five minutes faster, and decrease their obstacle course time each week of Second Phase. On top of the progressively difficult physical training, the number one priority of Second Phase is teaching students SCUBA (Self Contained Underwater Breathing Apparatus) diving. Students are taught two types of SCUBA: open circuit (compressed air) and closed circuit (100% oxygen rebreather). After Second Phase, students will be basic combat divers, with the physical ability to insert miles from a target and conduct several types of missions. This skill separates SEALs from all other Special Operations Forces.

Third Phase (Land Warfare)

Third Phase lasts for nine weeks. Demolitions, reconnaissance, and land warfare are the number-one priorities of this phase; however, this is also the most physically demanding phase of the three. Ten-mile runs, four-mile swims, and hundreds of pushups, pull-ups and situps must be done several times a week. Skills such as land navigation, small arms handling, small-unit tactics, patrolling techniques, rappelling, and military explosives are also mastered. This training is held at San Clemente Island and is classified. You'll have to get there before you learn any more about the highly physical and technical training of BUD/S Third Phase.

Running at BUD/S

To most BUD/S students, running is the most physically and mentally challenging exercise they will face. It is extremely important to have a strong running base before you arrive at BUD/S. If you do not, you will be one of the majority who become injured during the First Phase, and will have a greater chance of being dropped from the BUD/S program. Running up to four or five times a week at least three months prior to arriving at BUD/S is absolutely necessary. Chapter Five is devoted to teaching the proper techniques of running in the sand and preventing common overuse injuries.

P.T. at BUD/S

Upper body strength is a must at BUD/S. BUD/S PT lasts *at least* two hours and is conducted 3–4 times a week. These workouts can test even the seasoned athlete. TRUST ME; DON'T GO TO BUD/S IF YOU HAVE NEVER DONE THE EXERCISES IN THIS BOOK! You should be able do several hundred pushups, situps, and flutter kicks in a complete workout. Practice these NOW, before you get to BUD/S.

> **WARNING:** Some of these exercises (flutter kicks, leg levers, abdominal stretches . . .) have been proven and disproven in certain studies to be harmful to your lower back. Navy SEALs have been performing these exercises for over 30 years. Former SEALs in their fifties and sixties still perform these exercises—but do these exercises at your own risk!

Swimming at BUD/S

You will have two-mile timed ocean swims wearing fins every week at BUD/S. It is an absolute necessity to swim with fins prior to arriving at BUD/S. You have to strengthen your ankles and hip flexors by swimming with fins. There is no other way to prepare yourself, and the swimming will be extra challenging for you if you are not prepared. However, the biggest challenge to all BUD/S students is the water temperature—70 degrees in the summer, 55 degrees in the winter. It does not take long to become hypothermic in temperatures this cold. Ask any SEAL and he will tell you that getting used to being cold was the hardest part of BUD/S. Most of the students who quit say they do so because the water was too cold for them.

BUD/S Obstacle Course

The BUD/S "O-Course" is a test of upper body strength and cardiovascular stamina. The only way to improve at the O-Course is by constantly practicing. It will help if you climb ropes and do hundreds of pull-ups prior to arriving at BUD/S. Obstacles with ropes surrounded by soft sand will challenge anyone, but it will break a person who has slacked off on his upper body exercises. Climb ropes as often as you run—four to five times per week!

Final Comments About BUD/S

BUD/S is said to be the "toughest military training in the world." It is definitely challenging both mentally and physically. The instructors at BUD/S will make demands on your body for six months. You must be in the best shape of your life to succeed at BUD/S; but more importantly, you must be mentally focused and strong or you will become one of the 70–75% who drop out of training. The workout I designed will make you physically fit. If you have the desire to stick to this workout every day, by the end you might just have what it takes to succeed at BUD/S. You will definitely be physically prepared, but will you be mentally prepared? That is up to you.

This is what you must prepare yourself for:

First Phase	*Second Phase*	*Third Phase*
four-mile timed runs	four-mile timed runs	four-mile timed runs
up to one-mile swims	up to two-mile ocean swims	two-three-mile ocean swims
obstacle courses	obstacle courses	obstacle courses
50m underwater swim*	5.5-mile ocean swim*	15-mile timed run*
upper body PT	upper body PT	upper body PT
soft-sand runs	soft-sand runs	soft-sand runs
HELLWEEK*		

*Special one-time events. All other events occur WEEKLY!

How do you mentally prepare yourself for BUD/S?

First, being physically prepared will help you become mentally tough. Just as your endurance will grow each day with this program, so will your confidence. Knowing in your heart that you can complete the evolutions listed above without even thinking of quitting is the secret to excelling at BUD/S. For me, knowing that if I quit, I had to serve on a ship for the next five years was enough motivation. Others have something to prove to themselves, their family, or their friends. The key is to find what motivates you to succeed and then stay focused on that motivator when the days are long and the nights are just beginning. During Hell Week, take one hour at a time. Do not think that because you are exhausted and are only two hours into the 120-hour week that you cannot complete Hell Week. Instead think about making it to the next meal. Students get to sit, rest, and eat for almost an hour every six hours during Hell Week.

Cold Water

It will help if you become accustomed to ocean water, especially water temperature in the 60s. Ocean swims and body surfing are great ways to prepare yourself for the "Surf Zone." If you do not have access to ocean water, swim with fins in a pool for a couple of hours a few times a week. You have to realize that the BUD/S instructors can only keep you in the water for a certain period of time—NOTHING WILL LAST FOREVER.

Safety!

I do not recommend swimming alone in a pool, but especially not in the ocean. Navy SEALs always have a "swim buddy" with them no matter what they are doing. If you do not have a friend who shares your same desires and work ethic, at least have a lifeguard watch you swim.

Good luck—I hope you find what motivates you to never quit!

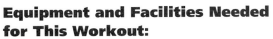

Equipment and Facilities Needed for This Workout:

- Access to a pool, either 25m or 25 yd, 50m or 50 yd.

- Access to a track or measured running area, 400m/400 yd.

- Access to pull-up bars and dip bars (parallel bars).

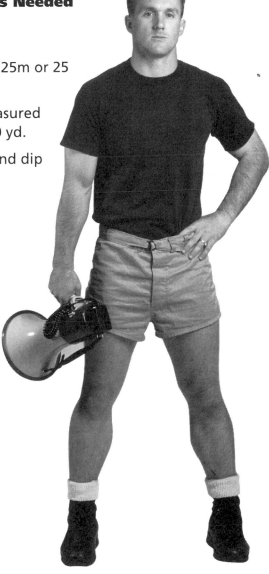

STRETCHING

The following stretches should be completed before and after every workout. Stretching will minimize or prevent the onset of muscle soreness due to rigorous physical activity. It only takes a few minutes to stretch (preferably 10 minutes before the workout and 10–15 minutes after you are finished). If you consistently stretch, you will minimize your risk of injuries, your muscles will feel less sore, and your flexibility will increase, thus helping to make you a faster swimmer and runner.

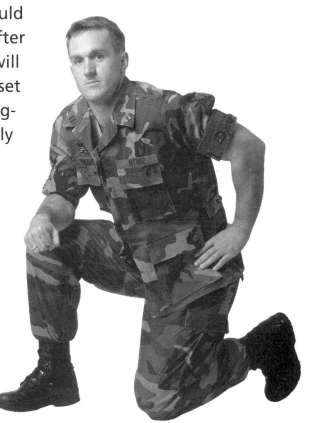

Stretching

Stretches	Repetitions / Time:
Jog	1/4 mile
Neck rotations	30 sec.
Arm and Shoulder	30 sec. each arm
Arm Circles	1 min.
Chest	30 sec.
Abdominal	30 sec.
Lower Back	30 sec.
Groin Stretch	30 sec.
ITB	30 sec. each leg
Thighs	30 sec. each leg
Toe Touchers	30 sec.
Calves	30 sec. each leg
Hamstring	30 sec.
Jumping Jacks	25 (4-count)

Neck Rotations

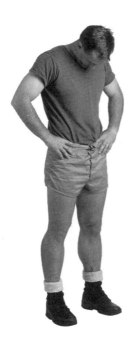

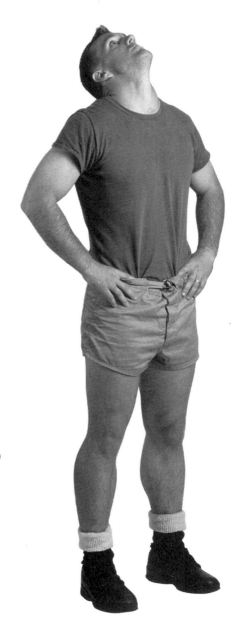

Front to back

Relax your neck muscles and move your head slowly up and down. Try to touch your chin to your chest on the down movement. Continue for 30 seconds.

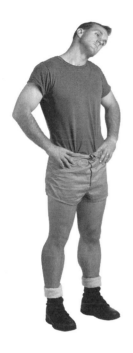

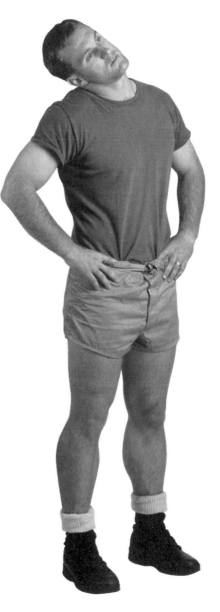

Side to Side

Relax your neck muscles and move your head slowly to the left and right. Move your head as if you were trying to touch your shoulder to your ear. Continue for 30 seconds.

Arm and Shoulder Stretch

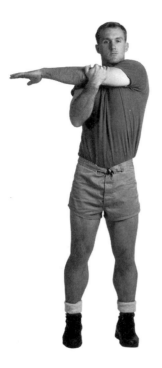

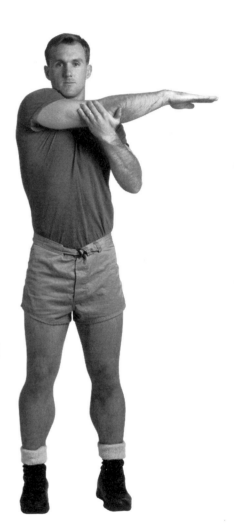

Arm and Shoulder Stretch #1

With your left hand, grab your right arm at the elbow and pull across your body. Hold for 15 seconds—switch arms.

Arm and Shoulder Stretch

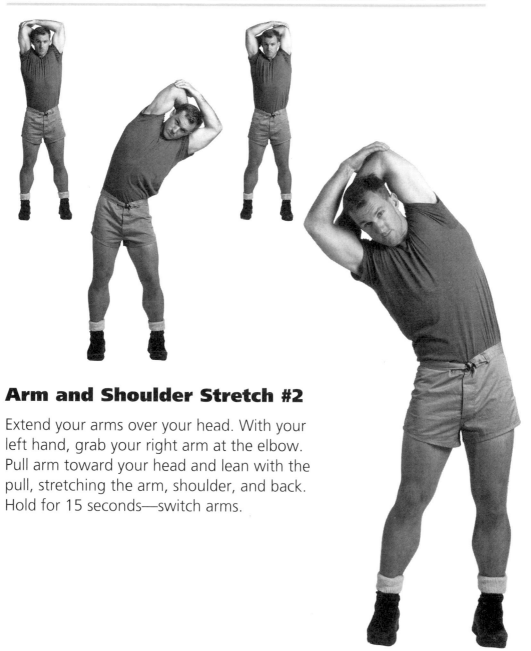

Arm and Shoulder Stretch #2

Extend your arms over your head. With your left hand, grab your right arm at the elbow. Pull arm toward your head and lean with the pull, stretching the arm, shoulder, and back. Hold for 15 seconds—switch arms.

Arm Circles

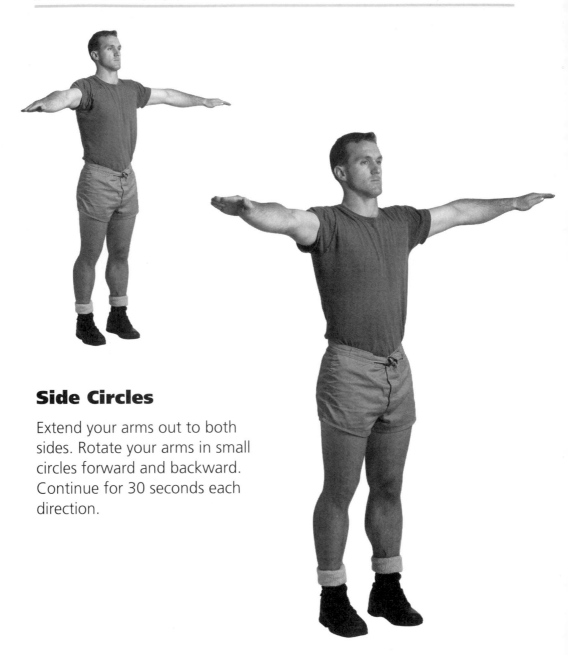

Side Circles

Extend your arms out to both sides. Rotate your arms in small circles forward and backward. Continue for 30 seconds each direction.

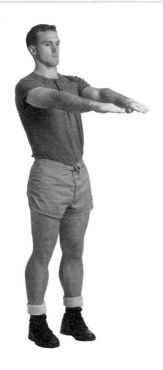

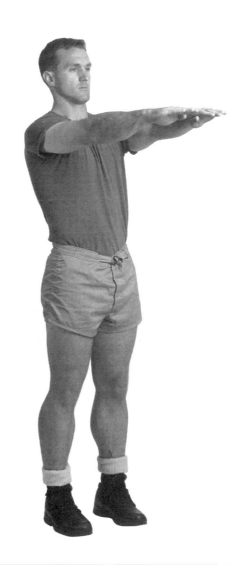

Front Circles

Extend both arms in front of you. Rotate your arms in small circles inward and outward. Continue for 30 seconds each direction.

Chest Stretches

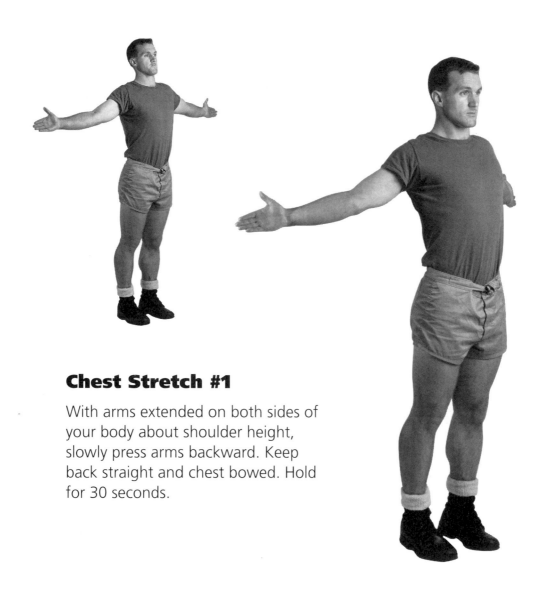

Chest Stretch #1

With arms extended on both sides of your body about shoulder height, slowly press arms backward. Keep back straight and chest bowed. Hold for 30 seconds.

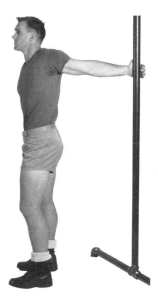

Wall Stretch

Place right arm on wall about shoulder height. Turn body away from the wall to the left. Hold arm in place. Hold for 15 seconds. Switch and repeat.

Abdominal Stretches

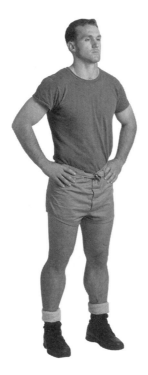

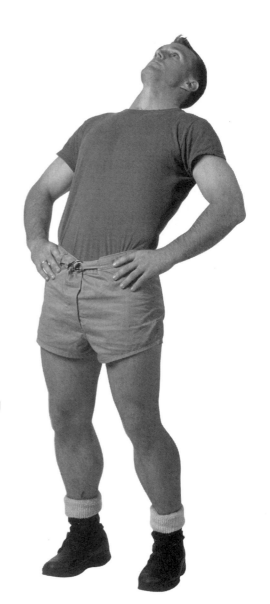

Standing

With your hands on your waist, slowly lean backward by pushing your hips forward and slightly arching your back. Hold for 15 seconds—repeat.

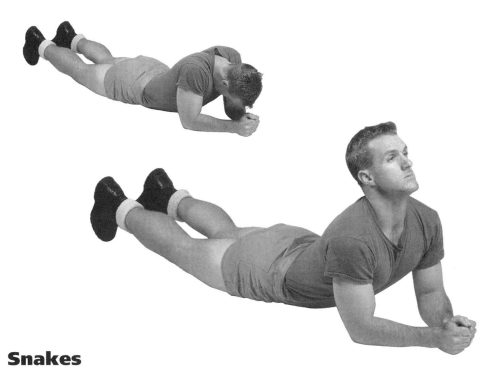

Snakes

Lay on your stomach. Place elbows under your chest and slowly lift your head and shoulders up, stretching your abdominal muscles. Hold for 15 seconds—repeat.

Lower Back Stretch

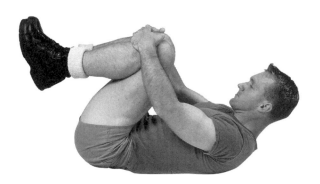

Chest to Knees

Lay on your back. Bring your knees to your chest and your head toward your knees. Hold for 15 seconds.

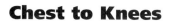

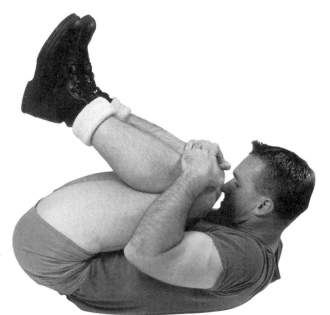

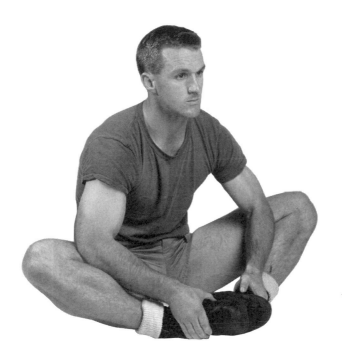

Butterfly

Sit on the floor with both legs bent outward and the soles of your feet touching each other. Grab your ankles with your hands and push down on your thighs with your elbows. Hold for 15 seconds—repeat.

ITB Stretch

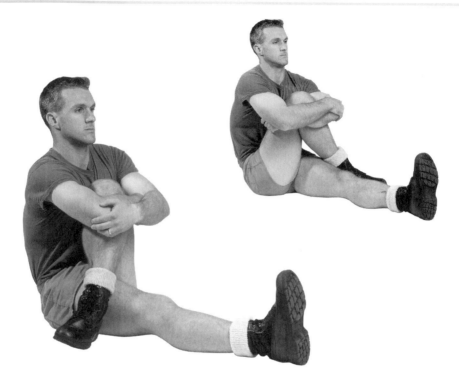

ITB Stretch #1 (Ilio Tibial Band)

Sit on the floor with both legs extended in front of you. Cross your right leg over your left. Bend and pull right leg to your chest and hold for 15 seconds. Switch and repeat.*

*Author's Note: Injury to the ITB due to overuse is very common among BUD/S students. For this reason, injury to the ITB is sometimes referred to as "I Tried BUD/S."

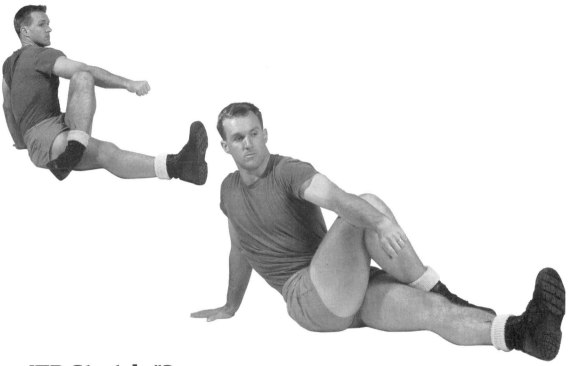

ITB Stretch #2

In the same position as Stretch #1, twist to the side of bent leg to stretch your lower back and ITB. Try to look in the opposite direction of your feet. Hold for 15 seconds. Switch and repeat.

Thigh Stretches

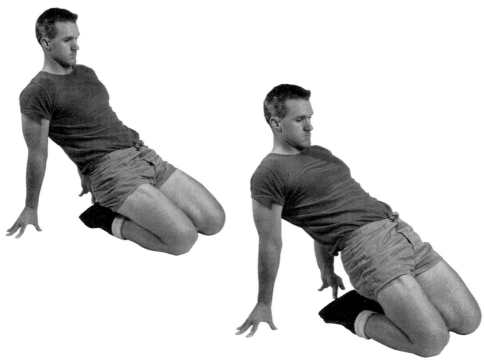

Sitting

Sit on your knees and heels. Lean backward so you can touch the floor behind you. Push your hips upward and hold for 15 seconds—repeat.

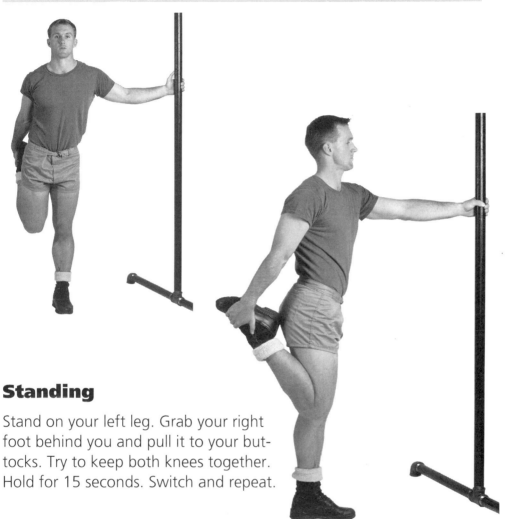

Standing

Stand on your left leg. Grab your right foot behind you and pull it to your buttocks. Try to keep both knees together. Hold for 15 seconds. Switch and repeat.

Toe Touchers

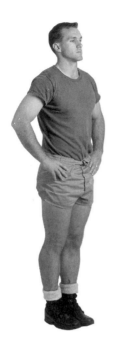

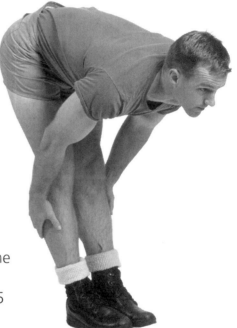

Standing or Sitting

With your feet together, bend at the
waist and grab the back of your
calves with both hands. Hold for 15
seconds—repeat.

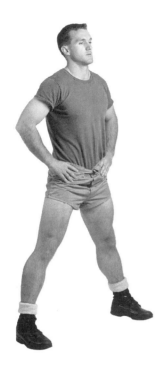

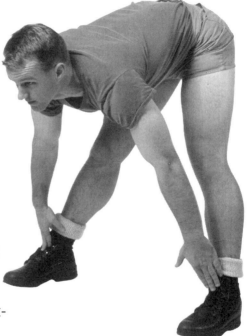

Standing or Sitting

With feet spread apart, bend at the waist and hold your back flat, stretching your hamstrings and lower back. Hold for 15 seconds—repeat.

Calf Stretches

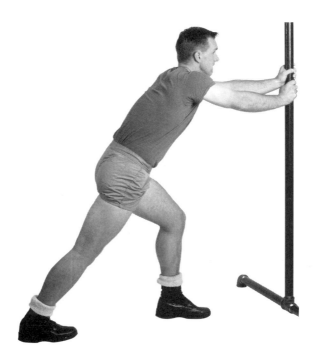

Gastrocnemius

Stand about four feet away from a wall or other sturdy object. With most of your weight on one leg, keep that leg straight and lean into the wall. Hold for 15 seconds—switch legs and repeat.

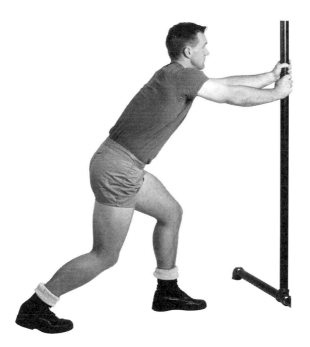

Soleus

Same stance as the Gastrocnemius Stretch, but bend your back knee slightly. You will feel the stretch in your Achilles tendon. Hold for 15 seconds—switch and repeat.

Hamstring Stretch

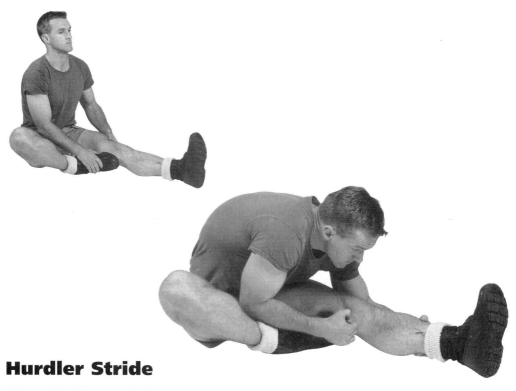

Hurdler Stride

Sit on the floor with legs extended in front of you. Bend right knee and place the sole of your right foot against the inside of your left knee. Grab feet and hold stretch for 15 seconds. Switch and repeat.

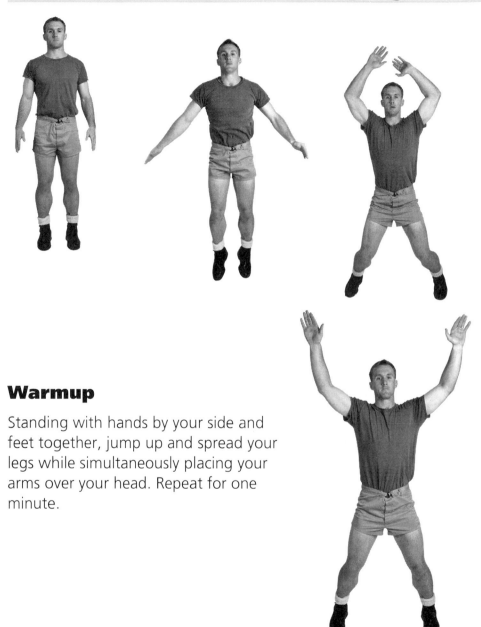

Warmup

Standing with hands by your side and feet together, jump up and spread your legs while simultaneously placing your arms over your head. Repeat for one minute.

P.T.

Physical Training, or PT, is a series of calisthenics and other exercises which are designed to strengthen your body. A combination of these exercises is referred to as "grinder PT" at BUD/S.

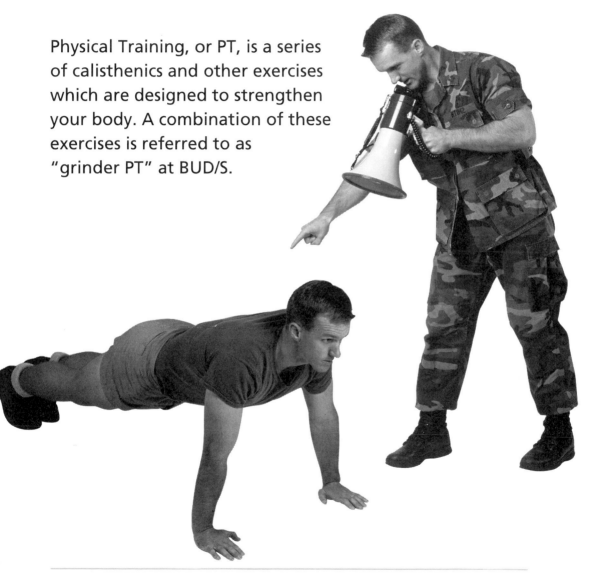

Upper Body Exercises

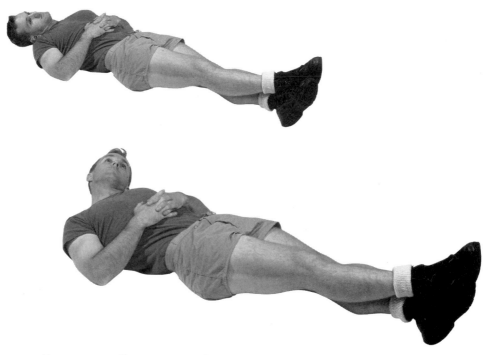

Neck Exercise #1: Side to Side

Lay on your back. Lift your head off the floor and move it from side to side for specified number of repetitions.*

*Author's Note: The number of repetitions for each exercise will vary depending on which day of which week of the program you are completing (see the 12 Weeks to BUD/S Workout chapter beginning on page 113). For example, in Week One, you will do 20 repetitions of the side-to-side neck exercise shown above. In Week Ten, you will do 100 repetitions of this exercise.

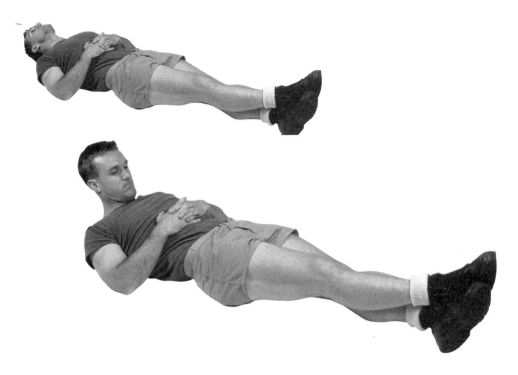

Neck Exercise #2: Up and Down

Lay on your back. Lift your head off the floor and move it up and down for specified number of repetitions.

Upper Body Exercises

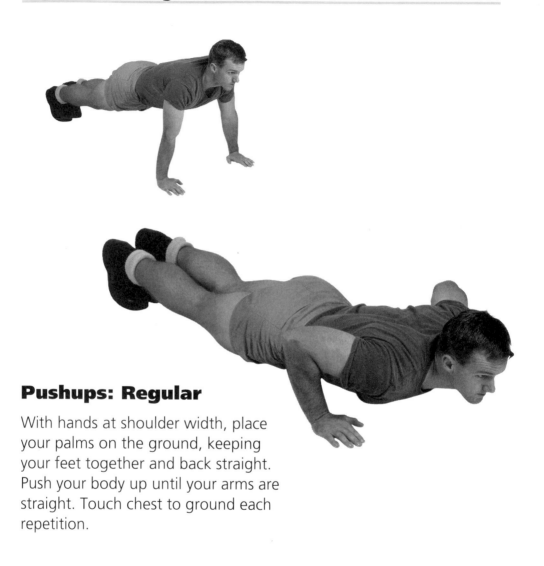

Pushups: Regular

With hands at shoulder width, place your palms on the ground, keeping your feet together and back straight. Push your body up until your arms are straight. Touch chest to ground each repetition.

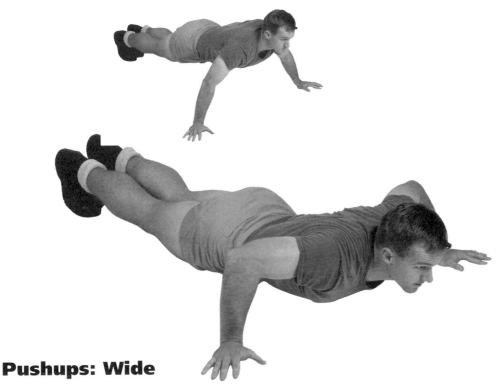

Pushups: Wide

With hands wider than shoulder width, place your palms on the ground, keeping feet together and back straight. Push your body up until your arms are straight. Touch chest to ground each repetition.

Upper Body Exercises

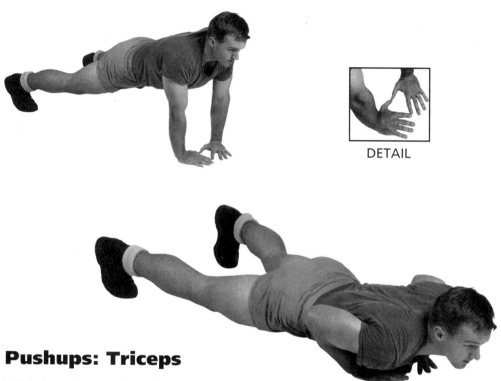

DETAIL

Pushups: Triceps

With hands touching, forming a triangle with your index fingers and thumbs meeting (as shown above), place palms on the ground, spreading your legs and keeping your back straight. Push your body up until your arms are straight. Touch chest to hands each repetition.

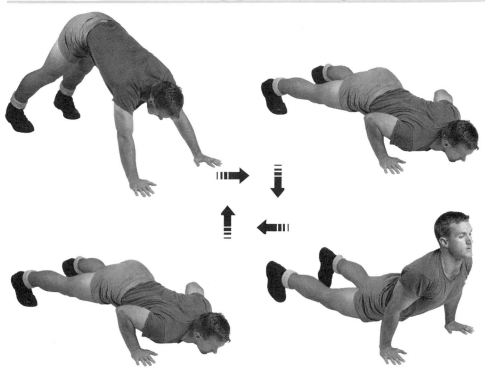

Pushups: Dive Bombers

Get into the pushup position, but bend at the waist and stick your buttocks in the air (Figure 1). Keeping your buttocks in the air, place chest to the ground in between your hands (Figure 2). Continue forward movement and push your chest through your hands and up by straightening your arms (Figure 3). Reverse the process and return back to starting position (Figure 4).

Upper Body Exercises

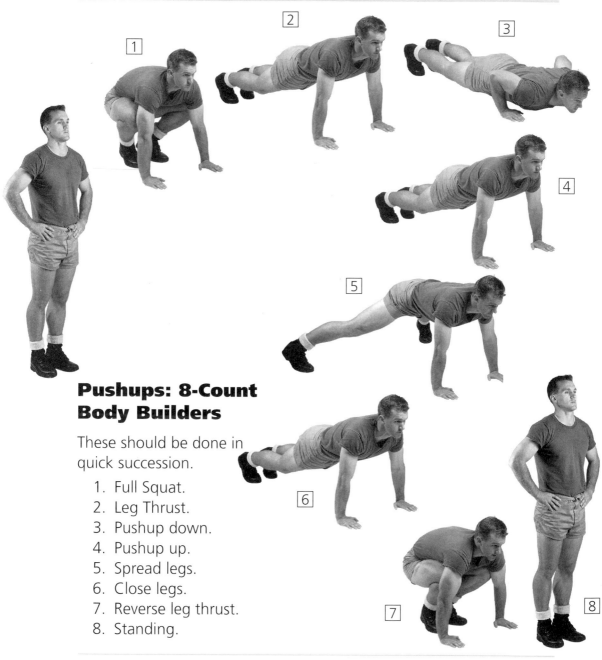

Pushups: 8-Count Body Builders

These should be done in quick succession.

1. Full Squat.
2. Leg Thrust.
3. Pushup down.
4. Pushup up.
5. Spread legs.
6. Close legs.
7. Reverse leg thrust.
8. Standing.

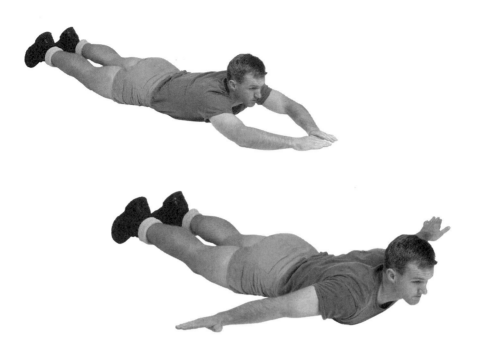

Arm Haulers

Lay on your stomach with your back arched slightly. Move your arms from the starting position over your head to your side (as if you were swimming). Keep your feet off the ground as well. This exercise works shoulders, lower back and buttocks.

Lower Body Exercises

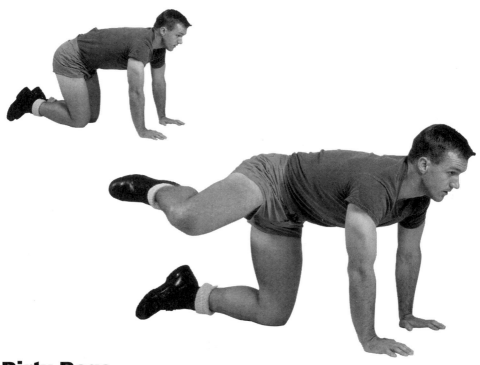

Dirty Dogs

Get into the "all fours" position. Lift your leg from your hip joint to the side for the specified number of repetitions. You may drop to your elbows for more comfort on your lower back. Switch sides and repeat.

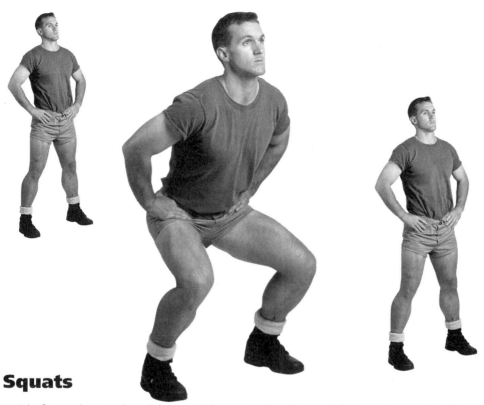

Squats

With feet about shoulder width apart, back straight, and eyes looking up, lower yourself by bending your legs almost 90 degrees at the knees. Slowly raise yourself after you have reached almost 90 degrees.

Lower Body Exercises

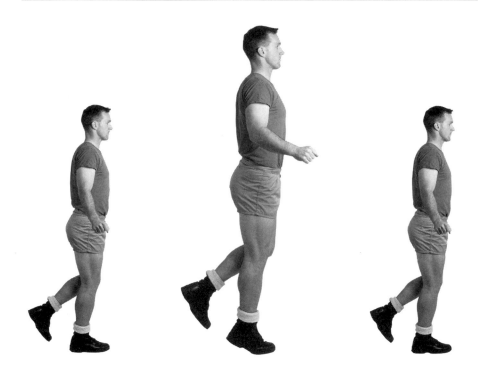

Calf and Heel Raises

Stand on one leg. Lift yourself up onto the balls of your feet by flexing the ankle joint and calf muscle. Switch legs and repeat for specified number of repetitions.

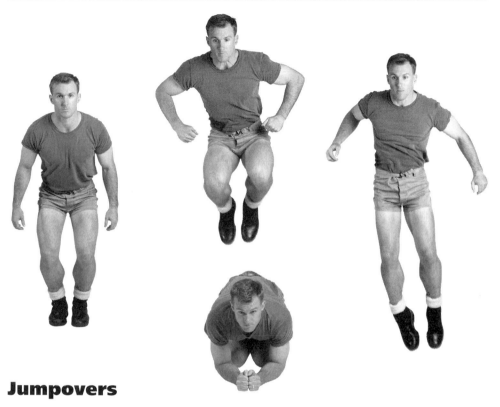

Jumpovers

Stand next to an object approximately 1.5–2 feet high. Jump from one side to the other for specified number of repetitions. Try to hit the ground on one side and jump back immediately after touching. Try not to double bounce.

Lower Body Exercises

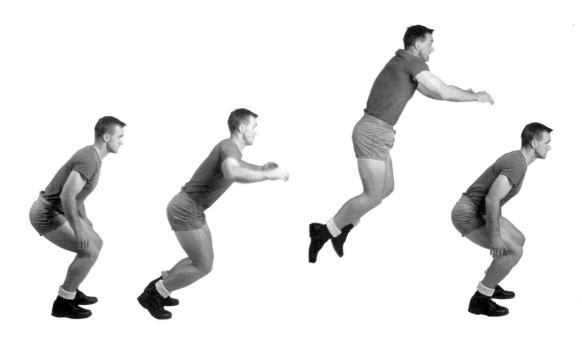

Frog Hops

From the squatting position, jump forward as far as you can. Repeat for specified number of repetitions.

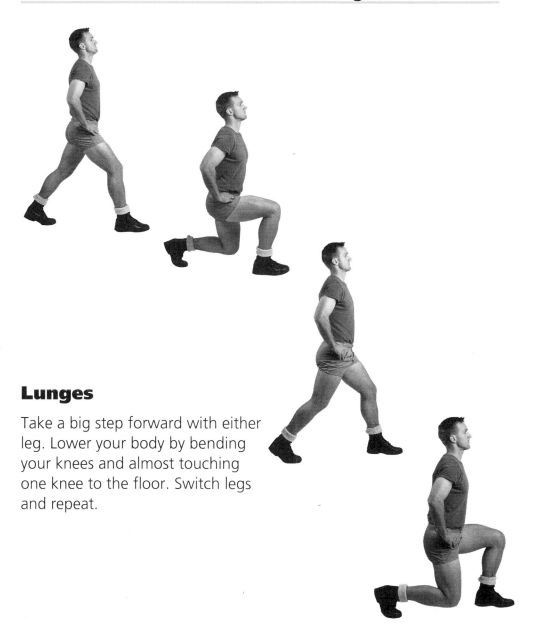

Lunges

Take a big step forward with either leg. Lower your body by bending your knees and almost touching one knee to the floor. Switch legs and repeat.

Abdominal Exercises

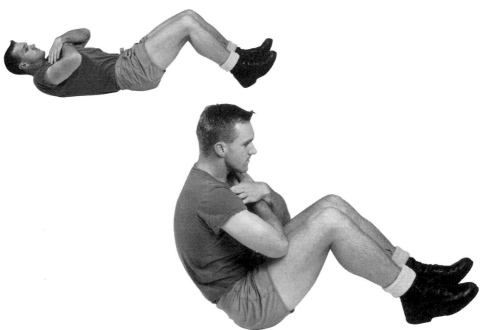

Situps: Regular

Lay on your back with your arms crossed over your chest and your knees slightly bent. Raise your upper body off the floor by contracting your stomach muscles. Touch your elbows to your thighs and repeat. Make sure you touch your shoulder blades to the floor each time.

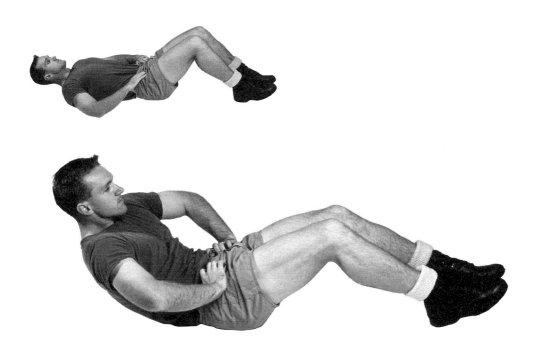

1/2 Situp

Lay on your back and place your hands on your hips. Lift your upper body so your lower back just comes off the floor, then slowly let yourself back down to the starting position. Repeat for specified number of repetitions.

Abdominal Exercises

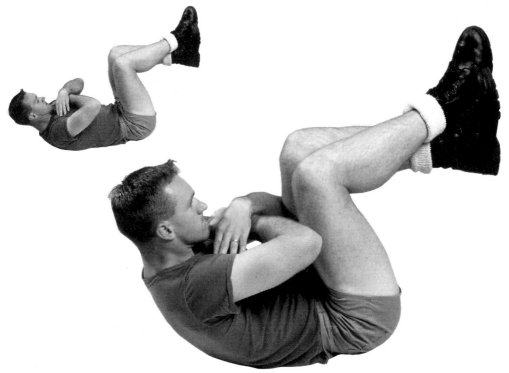

Crunches: Regular

Lay on your back with your legs up in the air and bent at the knees, forming a 90 degree angle with your legs. Bring your elbows to your knees. DO NOT PUT YOUR HANDS BEHIND YOUR HEAD AND PULL ON YOUR NECK.

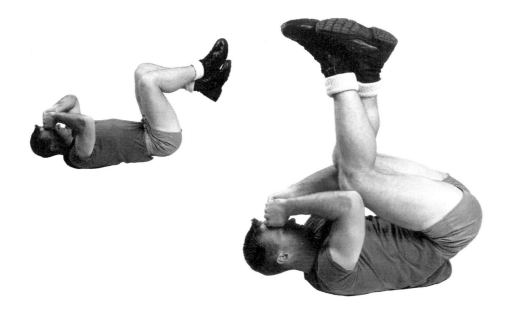

Crunches: Reverse

Lay on your back with your legs up in the air and bent at the knees, forming a 90 degree angle with your legs. Bring your knees to your elbows, lifting your lower back and buttocks off the ground. Keep your upper body still.

Abdominal Exercises

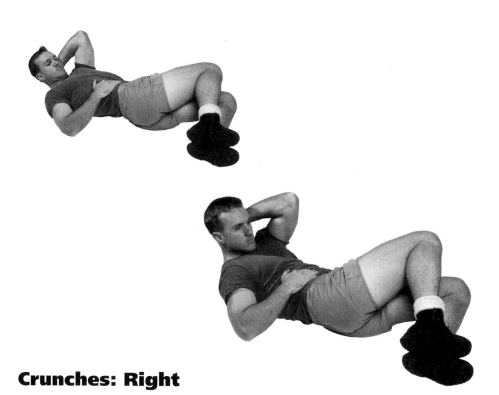

Crunches: Right

Lay with your shoulders and back flat on the floor, twisting your waist and legs so that you are laying on the left side of your hip. Crunch upward with your left arm and shoulder across your body toward the right side of your hip.

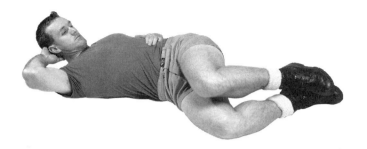

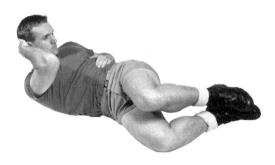

Crunches: Left

Lay with your shoulders and back flat on the floor, twisting your waist and legs so that you are laying on the right side of your hip. Crunch upward with your right arm and shoulder across your body toward the left side of your hip.

Abdominal Exercises

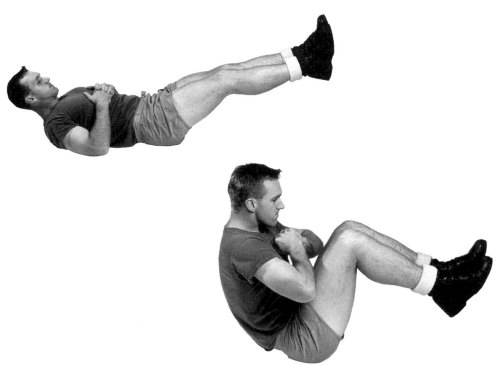

Situps: Atomic

Lay on your back. Lift your feet 6 inches off the floor and pull your knees toward your chest while simultaneously lifting your upper body off the floor.

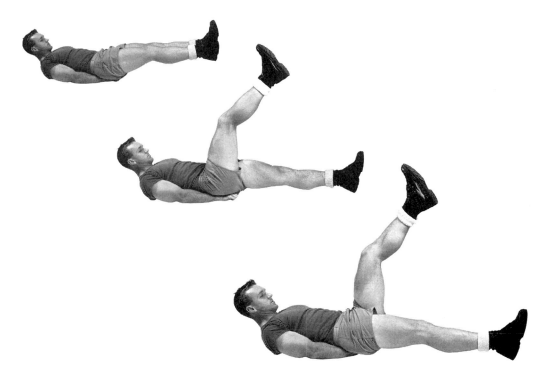

4-count Flutter Kicks

Place your hands under your hips. Lift legs 6 inches off the ground and begin "walking," raising each leg approximately 3 feet off the ground. Keep your legs straight and constantly moving. With each "step" you take, count 1, so the sequence will go as follows: 1, 2, 3,(1); 1, 2, 3,(2); 1, 2, 3,(3); . . . for the specified number of repetitions.

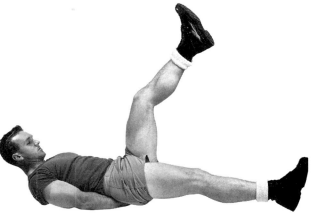

Abdominal Exercises

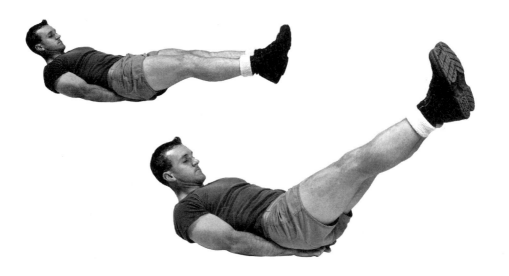

Leg Levers

Lay on your back with your hands under your hips and your legs together 6 inches off the floor. Lift your legs about 3 feet off the floor and slowly bring them down. Repeat. Do not let your legs touch the ground.

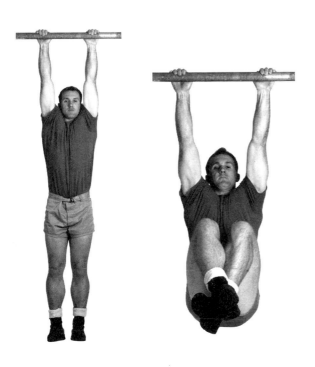

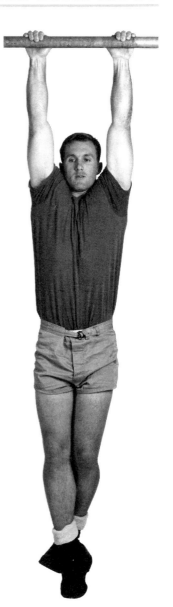

Hanging Knee Ups

Hang on a pull-up bar, as if you were performing a regular pull-up. Pull your knees as high as you can, trying to roll your knees into your chest.

PULL-UPS
AND DIPS

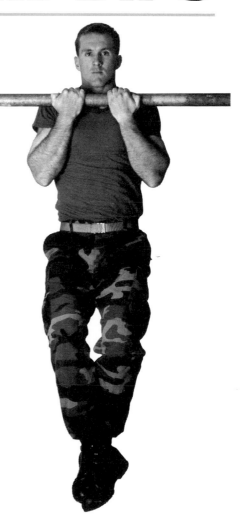

There are five different types of pull-ups which work various groups of arm and back muscles. The pull-up workout that requires sets of 2,4,6,8, and 10 repetitions for every type of pull-up is challenging, but offers moments of recovery and rest.

A Word About Pull-ups

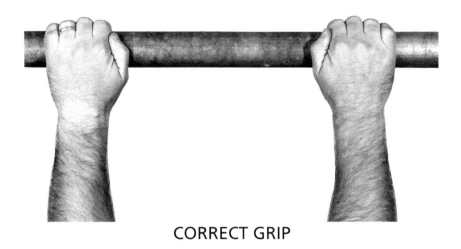

CORRECT GRIP

To strengthen your grip when doing pull-ups, make sure you use the correct grip shown above. This will increase the number of pull-ups you can do. Place your thumb next to your index finger and grip the bar with your fingers. Do not wrap your thumb around the bar.

A Word About Pull-ups

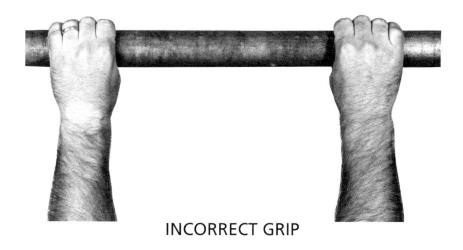

INCORRECT GRIP

The above photo, with thumbs and fingers wrapped around the bar, shows the grip that you should not use when doing pull-ups. With your thumb wrapped around the bar, your grip will weaken more quickly than if you use the proper grip shown on the opposite page.

Pull-ups

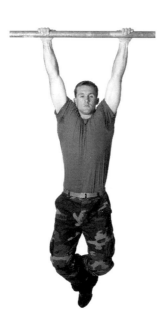

Regular Grip

With hands at shoulder width (see below), grab the bar and pull yourself up so your chin is lifted above the bar. Hold yourself above the bar for one second and let yourself down in a slow, controlled manner.

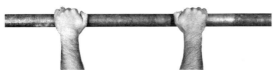

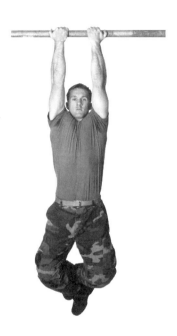

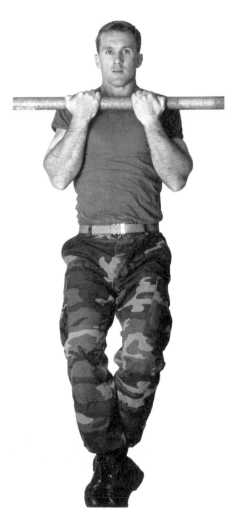

Reverse Grip

With your palms facing you (see below), grab the bar and pull your chin over the bar. Repeat for specified number of repetitions.

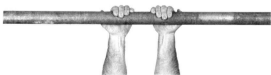

Pull-ups

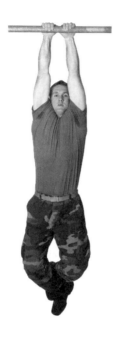

Close Grip

With your hands touching (or within 1 inch of each other), and palms facing away from you (see below), grab the bar and pull your chin over the bar. Repeat for specified number of repetitions.

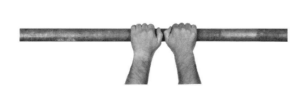

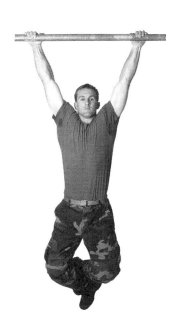

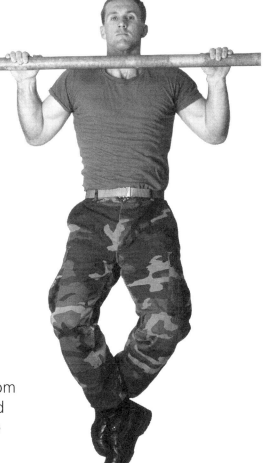

Wide Grip

With hands wider than shoulder width, and palms facing away from you (see below), grab the bar and pull your chin above it. Complete specified number of repetitions.

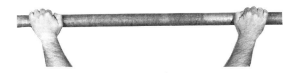

Pull-ups

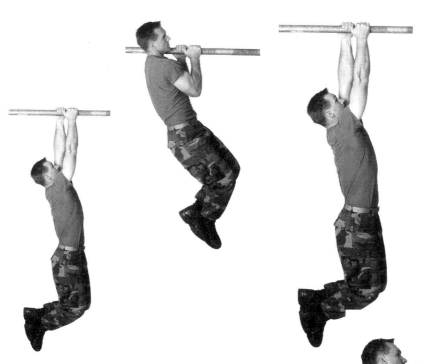

Pull-ups: Mountain Climbers

Place your hands together on the bar, one palm facing you and the other facing away from you (see below). Pull yourself up and touch your shoulder to the bar. Repeat, pulling yourself up on the other side of the bar.

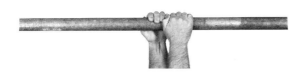

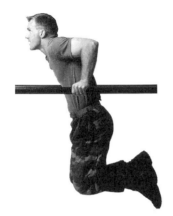

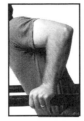 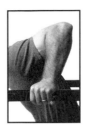

CORRECT   INCORRECT

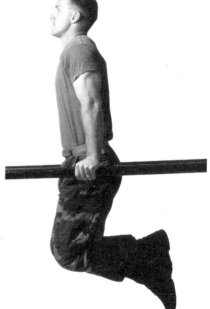

Bar Dips

Mount the two parallel bars with your hands on both sides of your body. Lift your body by straightening your arms. **Do not lock your elbows.** Slowly lower your body to a level where your arms make a 90 degree angle at the elbow joint. *Do not go lower than 90 degrees, because this is bad for your shoulder joints.*

RUNNING
AT BUD/S

Running in sand is more difficult than running on pavement, but less stressful on your joints. After several weeks of running in sand, your leg muscles will become stronger and you will have more stamina than ever before. Beach running is also an excellent cross-training tool to increase leg muscle definition, especially when you sprint regularly.

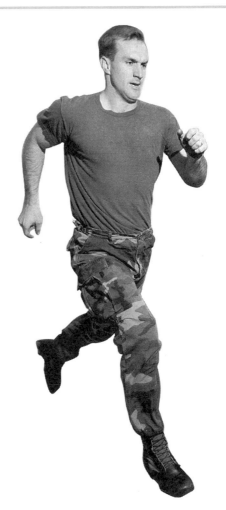

There is nothing quite like running in soft sand at BUD/S to challenge your desire to "never quit." It definitely helps to run on the beach prior to reporting to BUD/S because you'll need time to learn the techniques and adjust to the leg fatigue associated with soft-sand running.

To pass these runs, all you have to do is *stay with the pack*. Do not fall behind or you will be further tested through the formation of the GOON SQUAD. The GOON SQUAD is the group that does not stay with the pack on the platoon runs. If by the end of a run, a student is not back in formation, they will receive extra physical training in order to "motivate" them. A weekly four-mile timed run on the beach wearing combat boots is a test that will challenge even the best runners. Here are some training tips that will help you decrease your run times and stay with the pack.

Running on Soft Sand and Pavement

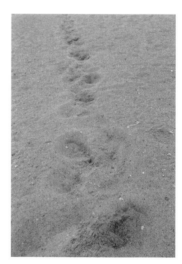

When running in the soft sand at BUD/S, **stepping in footprints** or previously made depressions is the biggest key to success. In soft-sand running, it is essential to change your stride to more of a shuffle and dig your toes into the sand. This will work your calves more than normal pavement running.

On pavement or hard-packed sand, **heel-toe contact** will help you with opening your stride and decreasing the stress on your knees and hips. Your foot should strike the pavement or hard surface with the heel of your foot and should roll forward across the ball and push off the ground with your toes.

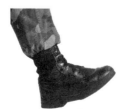 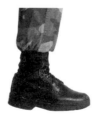 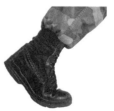

A good way to check your stride is the audible test. If you can hear your feet hit the ground, you are probably running flat-footed and need to open your stride. Shin splints and stress fractures soon accompany this unnatural style of running. So—run quietly!

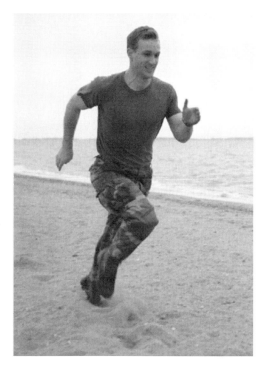

Regardless of the running surface, by far the most important technique of proper running is **breathing**. The proper breath is a very deep inhalation and exhalation. It should feel like a yawn. People who tend to take rapid, shallow breaths create carbon-dioxide build-up, increase their heart rate, and will encourage muscle cramps. Deep breaths get more oxygen to your muscles, rid your body of carbon dioxide, and aid in reducing fatigue.

Relaxing the upper body is another important running technique. When you are running, the only body parts that should be working are your lungs and your legs. If your upper body, fists, or face are clenched or flexed while running, the blood that should be going to your legs is sent to the flexed body parts as well, thus decreasing the amount of oxygen to your legs. Try to relax and breathe deeply.

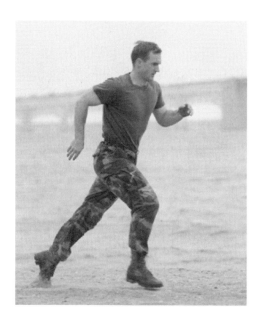 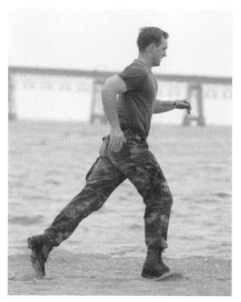

A **full arm swing** will help you get into a good running step and breathing rhythm. Your hands should swing in a straight line from your hips to your chest. Elbows should be bent slightly and hands should be loose and unclenched.

SWIMMING

The sidestroke, or combat swimmer stroke, is the trade-mark of the U.S. Navy SEALs. This stroke is used for stealth and efficiency. BUD/S students learn the basic stroke in a pool, without fins, and then advance to more chal-lenging environments such as the bay or ocean. The side-stroke is one of the easiest and most effective strokes you will learn. With the sidestroke, you have the advantage of being able to swim as far as six miles and still have the en-ergy to conduct a mission.

Sidestroke Without Fins

Swimming sidestroke without fins requires timing and coordination of kicks, arm pulls, and breathing. Preparing for the SEAL PFT 500-yard swim test will be easier if you follow the techniques and recommendations below:

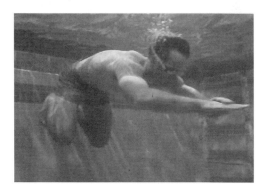

1. Kick off the wall. Every length of the pool, turn around, inhale, and kick off the wall, gliding until momentum almost stops. Start exhaling. Then, staying underwater, give one big double-arm pull and glide with your hands by your waist. Angle yourself toward the surface as you glide, because by this time you will need to breathe. When you break the surface to breath, you should be about 8–10 yards off the wall—with only minimal physical effort!

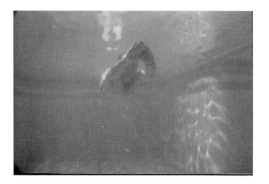

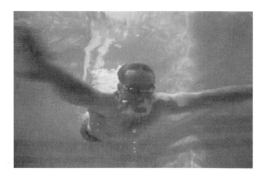

2. First breath. Turn to your side and extend your bottom arm over your head. Your top arm remains by your side as you pause for a big inhalation.

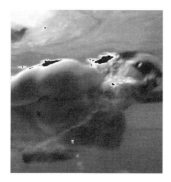 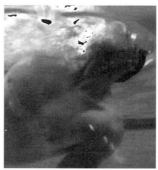 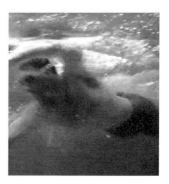

3. Pull and kick coordination. As your bottom arm begins its stroke and pulls toward your side (your top arm is already by your side), breathe, then move both arms over your head together. As your arms move forward, your top leg should also move forward as your legs spread to prepare for the big scissor kick.

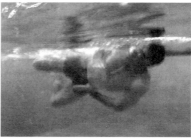

As you pull your top arm back to your side, kick and exhale at the same time. As your legs come together, the top arm should have completed its stroke and be by your side again as the bottom arm stays extended over your head. This is the glide position. Glide and breathe as you begin to pull your bottom arm to your side again.

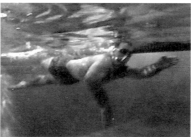

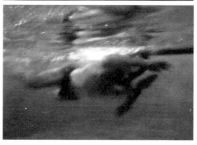

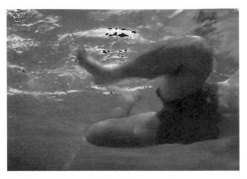 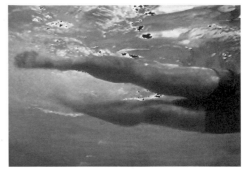

4. Flutter kick in between scissor kicks.

To help keep your momentum going and your body streamlined in the water, use 6-12" flutter kicks in between the powerful scissor kicks.

Sidestroke with Fins

You will use fins 99% of the time once you have entered the First Phase of BUD/S. Your ankles and hip flexors must be strong in order to do this; therefore, I recommend that you are able to swim at least one mile (with fins), without stopping, in less than 30 minutes before arriving at BUD/S. Sidestroke with fins is similar to the sidestroke without fins with only the following differences:

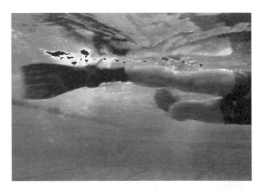

1. Constant flutter kicks.

With fins on your feet, your biggest source of power will naturally be your legs, so kick constantly in order to be propelled through the water.

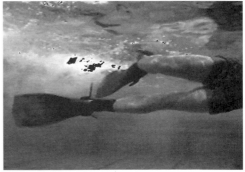

2. Swimming in a straight line. About every five to ten strokes, it is important to look forward in order to check if you are swimming in a straight line. This does not need to be done in the swimming pool; however, it is important in the open ocean to have a visual reference when surface swimming to check accuracy.

3. Arm pull and breathing coordination. As your top arm completes its stroke and the bottom arm is beginning its pull, breathe. When swimming with fins, your arms play an important role in getting your head above the surface to breathe, but can also be valuable in adding some power to your stroke.

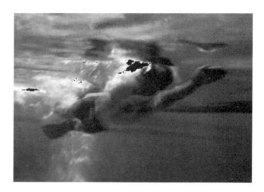

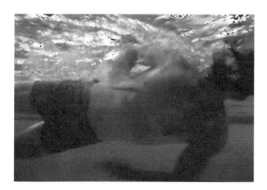

4. Recovery. As your bottom arm completes its stroke and is moving forward above your head, your top arm should be moving over your head just ahead of your bottom arm. Keep your top arm close to your body in order to reduce drag.

5. Stretch before you swim. It is extremely important to stretch your calves, ankles, and feet muscles/tendons before putting on your fins. You will lessen the amount of pain and fatigue in your feet and ankles if you stretch about 10-15 minutes before swimming over a mile in fins.

Crawlstroke (freestyle)

Hypoxic swim training. You will not use the crawlstroke much at BUD/S, but it is a great way to exercise and build your cardiovascular system, especially with hypoxic swimming workouts. The word **hypoxic** means low oxygen. Adapting this type of workout to swimming is easy, yet will probably be the most challenging cardiovascular exercise you will ever do. Hypoxic swimming easily compares to high-altitude training. Basically, your body is performing with less oxygen because of controlled breath holds while you surface swim. Instead of breathing every stroke or every other stroke, you will hold your breath for up to 10–12 strokes at a time. You will experience increased lactic acid levels, muscle fatigue, and an extremely high heart rate from hypoxic swimming, just as you would if you were running in the mountains. This gets your body used to performing with less oxygen, resulting in increased endurance when you swim regularly and breathe every stroke.

WARNING: Potentially dangerous—Do not perform alone!

Here are a few freestyle tips to help you increase your endurance and break up the monotony of sidestroke swimming:

1. Kicking off the wall. In pool swimming, kicking off the wall is essential to building up momentum and reducing the number of strokes per length. With your legs in a full squatting position against the wall, explode in the direction you are swimming and begin 6-inch flutter kicks. Keep your arms extended over your head. As your momentum decreases, begin the single arm pull, and surface to breathe. By this time you should be about 8–10 yards away from the wall.

2. 6-Inch Flutter kicks. Using 6-inch flutter kicks will help you maintain a streamlined position in the water by keeping your body position horizontal. Constant flutter kicks are not necessary, but are recommended for short distance and endurance swimming like you will be doing in this workout.

3. Arm pulls. An efficient arm pull is the most powerful and important part of swimming freestyle. The stroke begins with one arm extended over your head and ends when that arm is next to your hip. Each arm opposes each other and is never in the same position or moving in the same direction. As one arm is pulling through the stroke, the other is recovering forward.

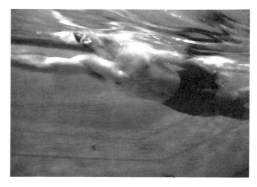

The arm pull is broken down into two parts: the **pull** and the **push**. As you pull one arm over your head, bend your elbow slightly and pull your arm under your body about 4–6 inches away from your chest. Once your hand is just below chest level, your pull stroke changes into a push stroke using the triceps muscles in your arm. From your chest, simply straighten out your arm until it brushes past your hips.

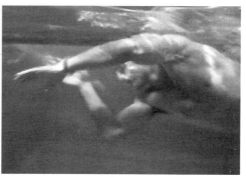

4. Recovery: Torso twist and high elbow. After a full arm stroke, recover the arm in front of you by getting your elbow high out

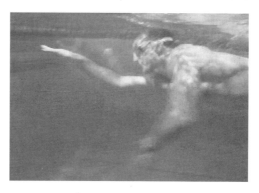

of the water. This is aided by slightly twisting your torso in order to get your shoulder and arm out of the water. Breathing requires you to twist your torso at the end of your stroke. Your hand should be by your hip with your other hand extended over your head. This enables you to slightly turn your neck to breathe while still, and most importantly, keeping your head in the water. Half of your face should still be underwater when you breathe. This is the most difficult part of freestyle to master—breathing and not lifting your head out of the water.

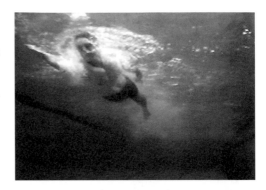

5. Keep your head down. Your body will act like a see-saw in the water. If your head comes out of the water, your lower body will sink, creating more drag and making your stroke much less efficient. A good rule of thumb is to make the water hit the hair line on your head as you glide through the water.

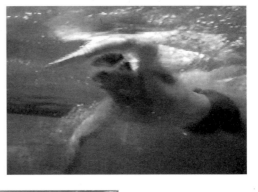

*The photos for this section were excerpted from the video Five Star Fitness Adventure: Navy SEAL Fitness: Preparing for the Teams. Techniques for mastering the sidestroke (with and without fins) and freestyle are detailed in full on this video, available from Five Star Fitness. For more information, please call 1-800-906-1234 or see the back pages of this book.

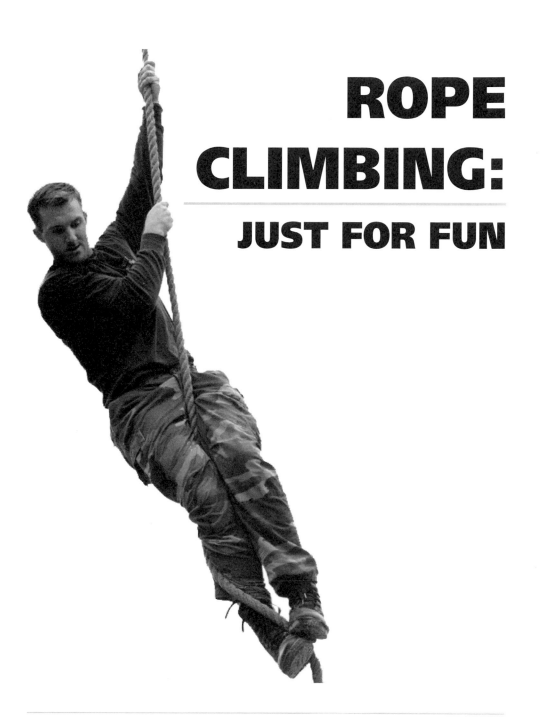

ROPE CLIMBING:
JUST FOR FUN

Basic Rope Climbing Techniques

Using your feet

Wrap the rope around your leg as follows: The rope goes at the inner thigh, between your legs, around your knee and calf on the outside of your leg, and across the top of your boot. With the unwrapped leg, clamp your foot on to the rope on your opposite foot. This will act as a brake and you can actually support yourself without using your hands and arms.

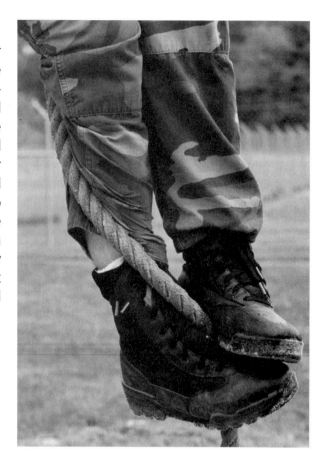

The technique to use so that you do not completely burn out your arms and grip is called the **_Brake and Squat Technique_**. Climb up the rope by bending your legs, sliding the rope across your foot by loosening the brake foot. Once you have moved about 1–1.5 feet of rope across your foot, brake and straighten your legs. Now you are using your legs to get you up the rope. This does require some amount of upper body strength but will save your energy for the most important part of rope climbing— GETTING DOWN!

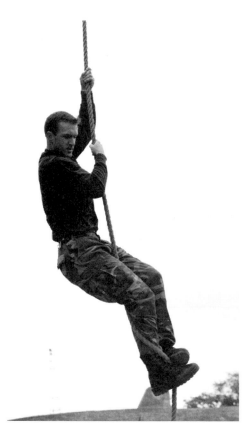

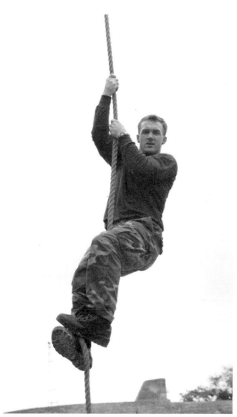

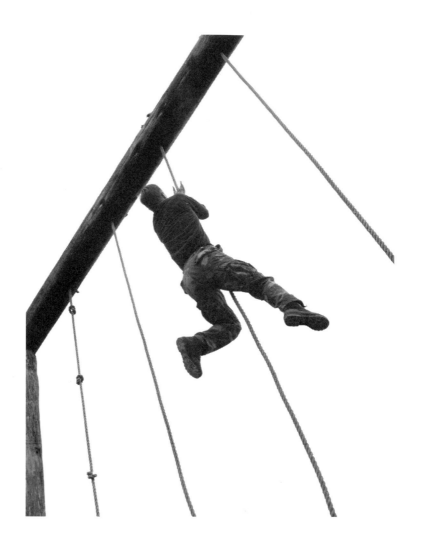

Advanced rope climbing—without your feet on the rope

This method of climbing a rope is a great workout and is absolutely exhausting. Your forearm muscles, biceps and back muscles will scream after a few times of climbing 30 feet of rope without using your legs.

Using a hand over hand method, slowly pull yourself up the rope about 6–12 inches at a time. This method requires an excellent grip (which you can first build by doing pull-ups) and biceps with stamina.

THE 12 WEEKS to BUD/S WORKOUT

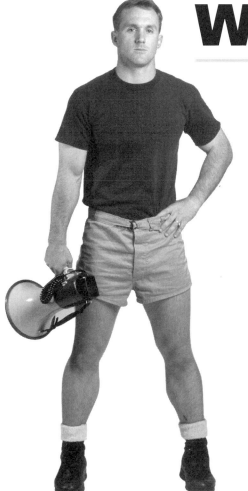

During the 12-week program, you will encounter many types of workouts. Each workout is designed to make you stronger in a different way. In the following pages, I've briefly explained each workout so you will have a better idea what to expect during your 12 weeks of intense exercising. In the course of the 12-week program, the structure of the workouts will stay the same, but the difficulty of each workout will grow as the number of repetitions increases.

The PT Pyramid

This workout is deceivingly difficult. The PT Pyramid is unique from any other workout because it has a warm-up, maximum, and a cool down period built into it. Begin climbing the Pyramid on the left side of the base. The levels of the Pyramid are the number of repetitions required in each set. Some exercises will have a (x2) or a (x3) next to the name of the exercise. The repetition number on the pyramid is multiplied by this number, making the workout much more challenging. Usually three or four different exercises are involved in this type of workout.

For example, the first sets of this workout go in this order:

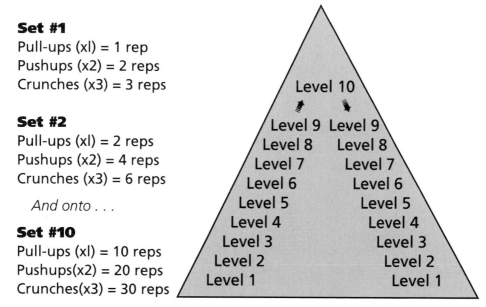

Set #1
Pull-ups (xl) = 1 rep
Pushups (x2) = 2 reps
Crunches (x3) = 3 reps

Set #2
Pull-ups (xl) = 2 reps
Pushups (x2) = 4 reps
Crunches (x3) = 6 reps

And onto . . .

Set #10
Pull-ups (xl) = 10 reps
Pushups(x2) = 20 reps
Crunches(x3) = 30 reps

Level 10
Level 9 Level 9
Level 8 Level 8
Level 7 Level 7
Level 6 Level 6
Level 5 Level 5
Level 4 Level 4
Level 3 Level 3
Level 2 Level 2
Level 1 Level 1

Once you reach the top of the pyramid, repeat the numbers and work your way down the right side until you are at the base of the pyramid again. Once you reach the bottom right side of the pyramid, you are finished. If you are beginning a workout program for the first time, do not go on to the following week's workouts until you can successfully complete the entire 19 sets of the pyramid workout.

Three-Mile Track Workout

The track workout is a great way to build speed and endurance for the 1.5-mile run as well as the 4-mile-timed run you will experience weekly at BUD/S. You will begin this interval training program by warming up with a steady one-mile run. This mile should be at a comfortable pace, usually a 7- to 8-minute mile. Run the next 1/4 mile at a full sprint; then jog another 1/4 mile at the same pace you ran the first mile. Repeat the 1/4-mile sprint and 1/4-jog again. Now repeat the same sprint/jog sequence with 1/8 miles four times, totaling another mile of interval training.

3-Mile Track Workout

1 mile jog (7:00–8:00 minute pace)	then . . .	1/4 mile sprint
1/4 mile jog (7:00–8:00 minute pace)	then . . .	1/4 mile sprint
1/4 mile jog (7:00–8:00 minute pace)	then . . .	1/8 mile sprint
1/8 mile jog	then . . .	1/8 mile sprint
1/8 mile jog	then . . .	1/8 mile sprint
1/8 mile jog	then . . .	1/8 mile sprint
1/8 mile jog		

This is not a walking workout. The object of interval training is to catch your breath from running while still moving at a jogging pace. This will speed your recovery time when you are resting. Quicker recovery time means you have more stamina and endurance, and will feel better after rigorous exercise than ever before.

If you have to build yourself up to the above workout by either decreasing the distance or speed, or walking during the jogging portion of the workout, that is fine! The object of this workout is to push yourself, but you can build a foundation by working your way up to the specified times and distances of the 3-Mile Track Workout.

Hypoxic Swim Pyramid

• Do not perform this workout alone •

The term hypoxic means low oxygen. By holding your breath and surface swimming (freestyle), you will receive a cardiovascular workout like no other. The only comparisons to hypoxic swimming are high-altitude running and cross-country skiing. The reason these workouts are similar is because exercise in high-altitudes, where there is less oxygen in the air, deprives your muscles of the oxygen you need. The same is true for holding your breath while swimming. Lactic acid and fatigue quickly build in your body as you exercise in low oxygen environments; therefore, you can get into much better shape in a shorter amount of time.

After training with a regimented hypoxic swim workout, when you swim normally (breathing every other stroke) your body will have become accustomed to not receiving sufficient oxygen. Thus, you will have more than enough oxygen to feed your muscles, and your performance will be greatly enhanced.

Run / Swim / Run

The Run / Swim / Run workout is one of the best ways to build the endurance you will need for SEAL training. This lower body, cardiovascular exercise program will enable you to build the stamina and endurance needed for increasing your Navy SEAL PFT scores. The object of this workout is to run the specified distance as fast as you can and quickly start swimming with little transition time. After swimming, immediately begin running again, and try to match your pace from the first run of the workout.

Swim-PT

The Swim-PT workout is a quick way to receive a great cardiovascular workout and build muscle stamina at the same time. The challenge of the Swim-PT workout is to swim 100 meters, jump out of the pool, and immediately begin performing pushups and abdominal exercises. After the pushups and situps are completed, jump back in the water and swim 100 meters. Repeat the above sequence for the specified number of sets.

Pull-up Workout

Here's how it works:

	Regular	Reverse	Close	Wide	Mountain Climber Grip
Set #	1–5	6–10	11–15	16–20	21–25
Reps	2,4,6,8,10	2,4,6,8,10	2,4,6,8,10	2,4,6,8,10	2,4,6,8,10
Total	30 reps +	30 reps +	30 reps +	30 reps +	30 reps =150 reps

The above workout is the most advanced pull-up workout of **The Complete Guide to Navy SEAL Fitness**, totaling 25 sets and 150 repetitions of pull-ups. Before you proceed to the next type of pull-ups, complete the 5 sets of 2, 4, 6, 8, 10 repetitions of the same type.

Super Sets

Most people have never done over 500 pushups and 500 situps in a 30–40 minute workout. Each set of six exercises should be completed within a two-minute period; therefore, the 20 super set workout should be finished within 40 minutes. For example, the 20 super set workout in week #3 is done the following way:

Set #1: 10 Situps ➡ 10 Pushups ➡ 10 Atomic Situps ➡ 10 Triceps Pushups ➡ 10 Leg Levers ➡ 10 Dive Bomber or Wide Grip Pushups

Repeat sequence 19 times.

The total number of pushups and abdominal exercises in this workout is 600 (each!). This workout is sometimes referred to as the "Time-Saver" workout. If you are running short on time, you can finish 300 pushups and situps in just 20 minutes. If you are a beginner, I recommend you cut the number of super sets in half. You will still get 300 repetitions in your workout, but it is important to build a solid base for several months before you attempt to challenge yourself with 600 repetitions of any exercise.

Lower Body PT

If you are not used to exercising your legs, you must stretch before, during, and after Lower Body PT. These exercises are explosive and plyometric exercises designed to build speed, strength and endurance. In this workout, you will concentrate on exercises such as frog hops, jumpovers, and lunges, designed to build the power in your legs. Whether you are running in boots on soft sand or swimming with fins in the ocean, you will need to have fit and strong legs. If you are not interested in SEAL training, Lower Body PT will build definition in your legs. Perform each exercise the specified number of repetitions, take 15 seconds to stretch, and repeat until all the exercises are completed.

Pushup / Situp / Dip Pyramid

The object of the Pushup/ Situp/ Dip Pyramid is to rapidly increase the repetitions in your workout. You will need to perform high repetitions at BUD/S and this is a great way to prepare for hundreds of pushups and situps. The workout goes like this: Begin with pushups and do 20 repetitions the first set. Then, alternate exercises and do 40 repetitions of situps. Next, quickly change to the dip position and perform 15 repetitions. Basically, you are climbing three pyramids at the same time, alternating exercises until you have reached the bottom right of all three pyramids. The toughest set is 50 pushups, 100 situps, and 30 dips.

Minimal Running Week

Statistically, lower extremity injuries occur during the third week of any running program. Overuse (too much running) or improper preparation will definitely result in injuries to your shins, feet, knees, and/or hips. You should take advantage of this week and stretch well, rest, and ice your joints and shins. You will not get out of shape because you are not running. This week will be challenging because of the amount of swimming you will do to replace the cardiovascular running workout. If you are 100% healthy and an advanced athlete, you may ride a bike for up to one hour in addition to the swimming. It is recommended that you give your legs a break this week, because you will not get a rest in the upcoming weeks.

Now you are ready to begin.

**Turn the page to face Week #1,
and the 12-week challenge . . .**

Week # 1

MONDAY	TUESDAY	WEDNESDAY
SEAL PFT	**Swimming**	**Running**
500yd swim: sidestroke or breaststroke pushups: max in 2 min. situps: max in 2 min. pull-ups: max (no time limit) 1.5-mile run: Run in combat boots and pants	200m warmup 500m sidestroke 3 x 100m sprints with 20 sec. rest 200m cool down	3-mile timed run (sprint 1.5 miles, jog 1.5 miles)

Week # 1

THURSDAY	FRIDAY	SATURDAY

Swimming

200m warmup
1000m sidestroke
200m cool down

Upper Body PT

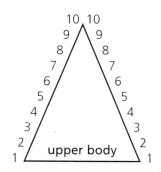

Pull-ups x 1
Pushups x 2
Situps x 3
each level of the pyramid

Neck exercises

up/down: 20
left/right: 20

8-count Body Builders: 10

Max pushups in 2 min.
Max situps in 2 min.
Max pull-ups

Running

4-mile timed run

Swimming

200m warmup
1000m sidestroke
200m cool down

Week # 2

MONDAY	TUESDAY	WEDNESDAY

MONDAY

Upper Body PT

Pull-ups	(sets x reps)
Regular grip	2 x 7
Reverse grip	2 x 7
Close grip	2 x 7
Wide grip	2 x 7
Mountain climbers	2 x 7
Pushups	(sets x reps)
Regular	2 x 15
Triceps	2 x 10
Wide	2 x 15
Dive Bomber	2 x 15
Dips	2 x 15
Arm Haulers	3 x 30

Neck exercises

up/down: 25
left/right: 25

Abdominal PT

Do two cycles of:

Regular situps	40
4-way crunches	40
(Regular, Reverse, Left, and Right: 40 of each)	
Leg levers	40
Flutter kicks	50
1/2 situps	40
Stretch 1 min.	

Running

3-mile timed run (sprint 1.5 miles, jog 1.5 miles)

TUESDAY

Swimming

200m warmup
500m sidestroke
3 x 100m sprints
4 x 50m sprints
200m cool down

WEDNESDAY

Upper Body PT

Pull-ups	(sets x reps)
Regular grip	2 x 7
Reverse grip	2 x 7
Close grip	2 x 7
Wide grip	2 x 7
Mountain climbers	2 x 7
Pushups (sets x reps)	
Regular	2 x 15
Triceps	2 x 10
Wide	2 x 15
Dive Bomber	2 x 15
Dips	2 x 15
Arm Haulers	3 x 30
8-count Body Builders	15

Max pushups in 2 min.
Max situps in 2 min.
Max pull-ups

Neck exercises

up/down: 25
left/right: 25

Abdominal PT

Do two cycles of:

Regular situps	40
4-way crunches	40
(Regular, Reverse, Left, and Right: 40 of each)	
Leg levers	40
Flutter kicks	50
1/2 situps	40
Stretch 1 min.	

Running

4-mile timed run

Week # 2

THURSDAY

Swimming

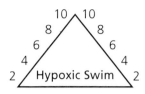

10 x 50m freestyle with 10 sec. interval (rest) in between each 50m (Each level of the pyramid is 50m.)

DO NOT SWIM ALONE!

Running

3-mile Track Workout
Jog: 1 mile in 7 min.
Sprint: 1/4 mile
Jog: 1/4 mile in 2 min.
Sprint: 1/4 mile
Jog: 1/4 mile in 2 min.
Sprint: 1/8 mile
Jog: 1/8 mile in 1 min.
Sprint: 1/8 mile
Jog: 1/8 mile in 1 min.
Sprint: 1/8 mile
Jog: 1/8 mile in 1 min.
Sprint: 1/8 mile
Jog: 1/8 mile in 1 min.

FRIDAY

Lower Body PT

Squats	3 x 10
Lunges	3 x 10
Frog Hops	3 x 10
Heel Raises	3 x 15
Jumpovers	3 x 15

Sprints

20m 1/2 pace x 2
20m full sprint x 2
40m 3/4 pace x 2
40m full sprint x 3
60m full sprint x 4
100m 1/2 pace x 1
100m full sprint x 2

Neck exercises

up/down: 25
left/right: 25

SATURDAY

Swimming

200m warmup
500m sidestroke
3 x 100m sprints (side)
4 x 50m sprints (side)
200m cool down

Running

3-mile timed run

Pull-ups   5 x 2,4,6,8 reps

Regular grip
Reverse grip
Close grip
Wide grip
Mountain climbers
Total Pull-ups = 100

Abdominal PT

Do two cycles of:	
Regular situps	40
4-way crunches	40
(40 each way)	
Leg levers	40
Flutter kicks	50
1/2 situps	40
Stretch 1 min.	

8-count Body Builders	15

Max pushups in 2 min.
Max situps in 2 min.
Max pull-ups

Week # 3

MONDAY

Swim/PT

10 sets of:
  100m freestyle
  20 pushups
  20 abs of choice

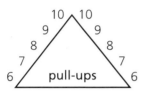

Dips: 25, 20, 15, 10

Neck exercises

  up/down: 25
  left/right: 25

No running: Due to common overuse injuries such as shin splints and stress fractures, take this week off even if you feel fine.

TUESDAY

Swimming

200m warmup
500m with fins
500m without fins
3 x 100m freestyle sprints
  at 1 min. 45 sec.
200m cool down

WEDNESDAY

Swim/PT

10 sets of:
  100m freestyle
  20 pushups
  20 abs of choice

Pull-ups 5 x 2,4,6,8 reps

  Regular grip
  Reverse grip
  Close grip
  Wide grip
  Mountain climbers

Neck exercises

  up/down: 25
  left/right: 25

20 Super Sets

Regular Situps	10
Regular Pushups	10
Atomic Situps	10
Triceps Pushups	10
Leg Levers	10
Dive Bombers or Wide Pushups	10

Do 20m cycles of all six exercises. You have 2 min. to perform each cycle. Total time: 40 min.

Week # 3

THURSDAY	FRIDAY	SATURDAY

THURSDAY

Swimming

200m warmup
500m with fins
500m without fins
3 x 100m freestyle sprints
    at 1 min. 45 sec.
200m cool down

FRIDAY

Swim/PT

10 sets of:
    100m freestyle
    20 pushups
    20 abs of choice

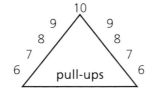

Dips: 25, 20, 15, 10

Neck exercises

    up/down: 25
    left/right: 25

SATURDAY

Running

3-mile timed run
(sprint 1.5 miles, jog 1.5
    miles.)

Swimming

200m warmup
500m with fins
500m without fins

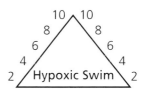

10 x 50m freestyle sprints
    at 1 min. 45 sec.
200m cool down

DO NOT SWIM ALONE!

Lower Body PT

Squats	3 x 15
Lunges	3 x 15
Heel Raises	3 x 15
Dirty Dogs	50

Week # 4

MONDAY

SEAL PFT

500yd swim: sidestroke or
   breaststroke
pushups: max in 2 min.
situps: max in 2 min.
pull-ups: max (no time
   limit)
1.5 mile run: Run in
   combat boots and pants

TUESDAY

Run-Swim-Run

Run: 3 miles < 21 min.
Swim: 1 mile with fins
   < 30 min.
Run: 3 miles < 21 min.
Total Time = 1 hr. 15 min.

Neck exercises

up/down: 35
left/right: 35

WEDNESDAY

Upper Body PT

Pull-ups 5 x 2,4,6,8 reps
   Regular grip
   Reverse grip
   Close grip
   Wide grip
   Mountain climbers
Total Pull-ups = 100

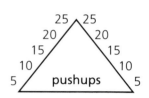

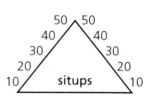

8-count Body Builders: 20

Max pushups in 2 min.
Max situps in 2 min.
Max pull-ups

Week # 4

THURSDAY	FRIDAY	SATURDAY

THURSDAY

Lower Body PT

Squats	10,15,20
Lunges	10,15,20
Frog Hops	10,15,20
Heel Raises	10,15,20
(each leg)	
Jumpovers	10,15,20
Dirty Dogs	100
(each leg)	

Neck exercises

up/down: 35
left/right: 35

Sprints

20m 1/2 pace x 2
20m full sprint x 3
40m 3/4 pace x 2
40m full sprint x 3
60m full sprint x 5
80m full sprint x 4
100m full sprint x 3

Swimming

200m warmup
500m sidestroke
500m freestyle
500m with fins
200m cool down

FRIDAY

Running

5 miles < 35 min.

SATURDAY

Upper Body PT

Pull-ups 5 x 2,4,6,8 reps
    Regular grip
    Reverse grip
    Close grip
    Wide grip
    Mountain climbers
Total Pull-ups = 100

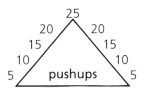

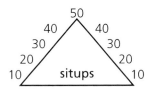

Neck exercises

up/down: 35
left/right: 35

8-count Body Builders: 20
Max pushups in 2 min.
Max situps in 2 min.
Max pull-ups

Swimming

2000m with fins

Week # 5

MONDAY

20 Super Sets:

Triceps Pushups	10
Regular Situps	7
Pushups	10
Reverse Crunches	7
Wide Pushups	10
1/2 Situps	7

Do 20 cycles of all six exercises. You have 2 min. to perform each cycle.
Total time: 40 min.
Total Pushups: 600
Total Abs: 420

Upper Body PT

Pull-ups: 16, 14, 12
Dips: 25, 20, 15
8-count Body Builders: 20, 15, 10

Neck Exercises:

up/down: 40
left/right: 40

Swimming

Swim with fins: 30 min.
Swim continuously for at least 1 mile.

TUESDAY

Run-Swim-Run

3-mile run
1-mile swim without fins
3-mile run

WEDNESDAY

Lower Body PT

Squats	3 x 15
Lunges	3 x 15
Frog Hops	2 x 10
Jumpovers	2 x 20
Heel Raises	3 x 20
Dirty Dogs	3 x 50

Sprints

20m x 5
40m x 5
60m x 5
100m x 4
200m x 2
440m x 1

Swimming

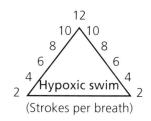

(Strokes per breath)

11 x 100m freestyle without fins. 15 sec. rest in between each 100m.

DO NOT SWIM ALONE!

Neck exercises:

up/down: 40
left/right: 40

Week # 5

THURSDAY	FRIDAY	SATURDAY

THURSDAY

Upper Body PT

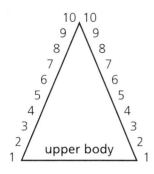

Pull-ups x 1
Pushups x 2
Abs of choice x 3
Dips x 2
Each level of the pyramid

Flutter kicks 100
Leg Levers 100
8-count Body Builders 25

Neck exercises:

up/down: 40
left/right: 40

Run-Swim-Run

3-mile run
1-mile swim without fins
3-mile run

FRIDAY

Swimming

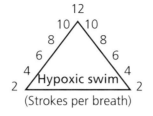
(Strokes per breath)

11 x 100m freestyle
without fins. 15 sec.
rest in between each
100m.

DO NOT SWIM ALONE!

Running

3-mile Track Workout
Jog 1 mile in 7 min.
Sprint 1/4 mile
Jog 1/4 mile in 2 min.
Sprint 1/4 mile
Jog 1/4 mile in 2 min.
Sprint 1/8 mile
Jog 1/8 mile in 1 min.
Sprint 1/8 mile
Jog 1/8 mile in 1 min.
Sprint 1/8 mile
Jog 1/8 mile in 1 min.
Sprint 1/8 mile
Jog 1/8 mile in 1 min.

SATURDAY

Upper Body PT

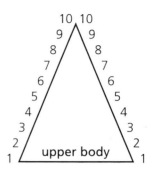

Pull-ups x 1
Pushups x 2
Abs of choice x 3
Dips x 2
Each level of the pyramid

Flutter kicks 100
Leg Levers 100

Neck Exercises:

up/down: 40
left/right: 40

Week # 6

MONDAY

10 Super Sets

Pull-ups	8
Pushups	20
Abs of choice	20
Dips	10

Abs Super Set x 2

Hanging Knee Ups	10
Regular situps	30
Oblique crunch	30
(left and right)	
30 each side	
Atomic situps	30
Crunches	30
Reverse crunches	30

Neck exercises:

up/down: 40
left/right: 40

Swimming

Swim continuously for 45
  min. with fins
  Goal: 1.5–2 miles

Running

4-mile Track Workout
Jog 1 mile in 7 min.
3 sets of:
  Sprint 1/4 mile
  Jog 1/4 mile in 1 min.
    45 sec.
6 sets of:
  Sprint 1/8 mile
  Jog 1/8 mile in 1 min.

TUESDAY

Swimming

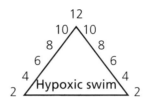

11 x 200m freestyle
without fins. 15 sec.
rest in between each
200m.

DO NOT SWIM ALONE!

WEDNESDAY

Lower Body PT

Squats	4 x 15
Lunges	4 x 15
Frog Hops	3 x 15
Jumpovers	3 x 20
Heel Raises	4 x 20
Dirty Dogs	2 x 100

Sprints

20m x 5
40m x 5
60m x 5
100m x 5
200m x 3
440m x 2

Swimming

Swim continuously for 45
  min. with fins
  Goal: 1.5-2 miles

Running

4-mile Track Workout
Jog 1 mile in 7 min.
3 sets of:
  Sprint 1/4 mile
  Jog 1/4 mile in 1 min.
    45 sec.
6 sets of:
  Sprint 1/8 mile
  Jog 1/8 mile in 1 min.

Week # 6

THURSDAY	FRIDAY	SATURDAY

THURSDAY

10 Super Sets

Pull-ups	8
Pushups	20
Abs of choice	20
Dips	10

8-count Body Builders: 5
Max pushups in 2 min.
Max situps in 2 min.
Max pull-ups

Neck exercises:

up/down: 40
left/right: 40

Abs Super Set x 2

Hanging Knee Ups	10
Regular situps	30
Oblique crunch	30
(left and right)	
30 each side	
Atomic situps	30
Crunches	30
Reverse crunches	30

Swimming

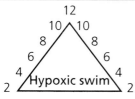

11 x 150m freestyle without fins. 15 sec. rest in between each 200m.

FRIDAY

Swimming

Swim continuously for 45 min. with fins.
  Goal: 1.5-2 miles

SATURDAY

Upper Body PT

Pull-ups: 4 x 2,4,6,8,10
  Regular grip
  Reverse grip
  Close grip
  Wide grip

Pushups: 50,40,30,20,10
Dips: 30,25,20,15,10
8-count Body Builders:
  25,20,15,10

Max pushups in 2 min.
Max situps in 2 min.
Max pull-ups

Neck exercises:

up/down: 40
left/right: 40

Abs Super Set x 2

Flutter kicks 100
Leg Levers 100
Situps 100

Week # 7

MONDAY

SEAL PFT

500yd swim: sidestroke or
   breaststroke
pushups: max in 2 min.
situps: max in 2 min.
pull-ups: max (no time
   limit)
1.5 mile run: Run in
   combat boots and
   pants

TUESDAY

Run-Swim-Run

Run 4 miles
Swim 3000m with fins
Run 3 miles

Lower Body PT

Squats	3 x 15
Lunges	3 x 15
Frog Hops	2 x 10
Jumpovers	2 x 20
Heel Raises	3 x 20
Dirty Dogs	3 x 50

Neck exercises:

up/down: 50
left/right: 50

WEDNESDAY

Swimming

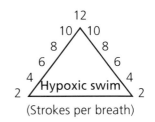

(Strokes per breath)

11 x 200m freestyle
   without fins. 15 sec.
   rest in between each
   200m.

DO NOT SWIM ALONE!

Week # 7

THURSDAY	FRIDAY	SATURDAY

Upper Body PT

Pull-ups :
Regular grip	2 x 7
Reverse grip	2 x 7
Close grip	2 x 7
Wide grip	2 x 7
Mountain climbers	2 x 7

Pushups:
Regular	2 x 30
Triceps	2 x 20
Wide	2 x 30
Dive Bomber	2 x 30

Dips	2 x 25
Arm Haulers	3 x 50

8-count
Body Builders	2 x 20

Max pushups in 2 min.
Max situps in 2 min.
Max pull-ups

Neck exercises

up/down: 50
left/right: 50

Abs Super Set x 2:

Regular situps	60
4-way crunches	50
Leg levers	60
Flutter kicks	150
1/2 situps	100
Stretch 1 min.	

Running

5-mile timed run

Swimming

1 mile swim with fins

Running

Run 6 miles.

Run-Swim/PT-Run

Run 4 miles.
15 sets: Swim /PT
  20 pushups
  20 abs of choice
  100m swim
Run 3 miles.

The Complete Guide to Navy SEAL Fitness

Week # 8

MONDAY

Upper Body PT

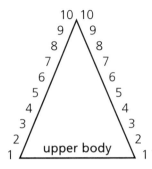

Pull-ups x 1
Pushups x 3
Abs of choice x 5
Dips x 2

Run-Swim-Run

Run 4 miles.
Swim 1 mile with fins.
Run 3 miles.

Neck exercises:

up/down: 2 x 35
left/right: 2 x 35

TUESDAY

Lower Body PT

Squats	4 x 20
Lunges	4 x 20
Frog Hops	3 x 20
Jumpovers	3 x 20
Heel Raises	4 x 20
Dirty Dogs	2 x 100

Running

4-mile Track Workout
Jog 1 mile in 7 min.
3 sets of:
Sprint 1/4 mile in 1 min. 20 sec.
Jog 1/4 mile in 1 min. 45 sec.
6 sets of:
Sprint 1/8 mile in 40 sec.
Jog 1/8 mile in 1 min.

Swimming

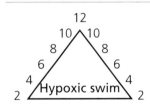

11 x 200m freestyle without fins. 15 sec. rest in between each 200m.

DO NOT SWIM ALONE!

WEDNESDAY

Swimming

Swim with fins 1.5 mile.

Neck exercises

up/down: 2 x 35
left/right: 2 x 35

Week # 8

THURSDAY	FRIDAY	SATURDAY

THURSDAY

Run-Swim/PT-Run

Run 3 miles.
10 Sets: Swim/PT
   100m sprints
   25 pushups
   25 abs of choice
Run 3 miles.

Max pushups in 2 min.
Max situps in 2 min.
Max pull-ups

FRIDAY

Upper Body PT

Pull-ups: 5 x 2,4,6,8,10
   Regular grip
   Reverse grip
   Close grip
   Wide grip
   Mountain climber
Total Pull-ups: 150

Arm Haulers: 2 x 75

Neck exercises:

   up/down: 2 x 35
   left/right: 2 x 35

Abs Super Set

Flutter kicks 150
Leg Levers 150
Situps 150

Swimming

Swim with fins 1.5 miles.

Running

Run 4 miles in 27 min, in
   sand if available.

SATURDAY

Running

Run 6 miles within 40 min.

Upper Body PT

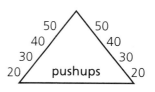

pushups: 50 50 40 40 30 30 20 20

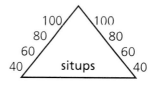

situps: 100 100 80 80 60 60 40 40

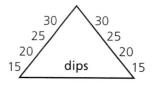

dips: 30 30 25 25 20 20 15 15

The Complete Guide to Navy SEAL Fitness

Week # 9

MONDAY

Upper Body PT

Pull-ups: 5 x 2,4,6,8,10
    Regular grip
    Reverse grip
    Close grip
    Wide grip
    Mountain climber

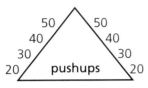

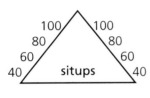

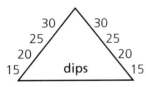

Arm Haulers: 2 x 75

Neck exercises:

    up/down: 2 x 40
    left/right: 2 x 40

Run-Swim-Run

Run 4 miles.
Swim 1 mile with fins.
Run 3 miles.

TUESDAY

Lower Body PT

Squats	4 x 20
Lunges	4 x 20
Frog Hops	3 x 20
Jumpovers	3 x 20
Heel Raises	4 x 20
Dirty Dogs	2 x 100

Sprints

20m x 5
40m x 5
60m x 5
100m x 5
200m x 3
440m x 2

Swimming

200m warmup
500m pulls (no kick)
300m kicks (no pull)
8 x 50m sprints
    (15 sec. rest between
    each)
2 x 100m sprints
    (20 sec. rest between
    each)
Hypoxic: 4,6,8,10
    (strokes/breath) x 100m
200m cool down

WEDNESDAY

Run-Swim-Run

Run 4 miles.
Swim 1 mile with fins.
Run 4 miles.

Neck exercises

    up/down: 2 x 40
    left/right: 2 x 40

Week # 9

THURSDAY	FRIDAY	SATURDAY

Swimming

200m warmup
500m pulls (no kick)
300m kicks (no pull)
8 x 50m sprints
  (15 sec. rest between
  each)
2 x 100m sprints
  (20 sec. rest between
  each)
Hypoxic: 4,6,8,10
  (strokes/breath) x 100m
200m cool down

Lower Body PT

Squats	4 x 20
Lunges	4 x 20
Frog Hops	3 x 20
Jumpovers	3 x 20
Heel Raises	4 x 20
Dirty Dogs	2 x 100

Running

Run 4 miles in 27 min.

Swimming

Swim 2000m with fins.

Upper Body PT

Pull-ups: 5 x 2,4,6,8,10
  Regular grip
  Reverse grip
  Close grip
  Wide grip
  Mountain climbers

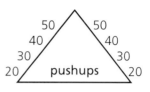

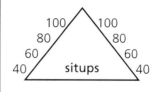

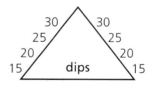

Neck exercises

  up/down: 2 x 40
  left/right: 2 x 40

Running

3-mile timed run.
(sprint 1.5 mile, jog 1.5
  mile)

The Complete Guide to Navy SEAL Fitness

Week # 10

MONDAY

SEAL PFT

500yd swim: sidestroke or
    breaststroke
pushups: max in 2 min.
situps: max in 2 min.
pull-ups: max (no time
    limit)
1.5 mile run: Run in
    combat boots and pants

TUESDAY

Running

Run 4 miles in 27 min.

WEDNESDAY

Upper Body PT

Pull-ups: 2,4,6,8,10 x 5
    Regular grip
    Reverse grip
    Close grip
    Wide grip

Arm Haulers: 2 x 75

20 Super Sets

Situps	10
Pushups	10
Atomic situps	10
Triceps	10
Leg Levers	10
Dive Bombers 10	

Run-Swim-Run

Run 3 miles.
Swim 1 mile with fins.
Run 3 miles.

Week # 10

THURSDAY

Lower Body PT

Squats	3 x 20
Lunges	3 x 20
Frog Hops	3 x 15
Jumpovers	3 x 20
Heel Raises	3 x 20
Dirty Dogs	2 x 100

Sprints

20m x 5
40m x 5
60m x 5
100m x 5
200m x 3
440m x 2

FRIDAY

Running

Run 5 miles in 33 min.

SATURDAY

Swim/PT

15 sets of:
    Freestyle sprints: 100m
    Pushups: 15
    Abs of choice: 15

Max pushups in 2 min.
Max situps in 2 min.
Max pull-ups

Arm Haulers: 2 x 75

Swimming

Swim 2 miles with fins.

Week # 11

MONDAY

Upper Body PT

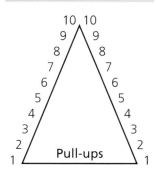

10 10
9   9
8   8
7   7
6   6
5   5
4   4
3   3
2   2
1   Pull-ups   1

25 Super Sets

Situps	10
Pushups	10
Atomic situps	10
Triceps	10
Leg Levers	10
Dive Bombers	10

Neck exercises:

up/down: 2 x 50
left/right: 2 x 50

Swimming

1-mile swim with fins

TUESDAY

Running

4-mile timed run

WEDNESDAY

Swim/PT

Hypoxic swim
5 x 50 at 50 sec. intervals
(6 strokes/breath)
4 x 50 at 55 sec. intervals
(8 strokes/breath)
3 x 50 at 1 min. intervals
(10 strokes/breath)
2 x 50 at 1 min. intervals
(12 strokes/breath)
1 x 50 (no breaths)

DO NOT DO ALONE!

Swim PT

10 Sets of:
100m sprint (freestyle)
15 pushups
15 abs of choice

Neck exercises:

up/down: 2 x 50
left/right: 2 x 50

Week # 11

THURSDAY

Running

4-mile timed run

FRIDAY

Swimming

1-mile swim with fins

Upper Body PT

Pull-ups: 5 x 2,4,6,8,10
  Regular grip
  Reverse grip
  Close grip
  Wide grip

Arm Haulers: 2 x 75

Neck exercises:

  up/down: 2 x 50
  left/right: 2 x 50

20 Super Sets

Situps	10
Pushups	10
Atomic situps	10
Triceps	10
Leg Levers	10
Dive Bombers	10

SATURDAY

Running

3-mile timed run
  (sprint 1.5 mile, jog 1.5
  mile)

Week # 12

MONDAY

20 Super Sets

Triceps Pushups	10
Regular Situps	7
Regular Pushups	10
Reverse Crunches	7
Wide Pushups	10
1/2 Situps	7

Total Time: 40 min.
Total Pushups: 600
Total Abs: 420

Pull-ups: 16, 14, 12
Dips: 25, 20, 15

Running

4-mile timed run

TUESDAY

Swimming

Hypoxic swim
  5 x 50m,
     50 sec. intervals
  4 x 50m,
     55 sec. intervals
  3 x 50m,
     1 min. intervals
  2 x 50m,
     1 min. intervals
  1 x 50m

DO NOT SWIM ALONE!

The number of breaths per
  50m = number of times
  you swim the 50m; ie, 5
  x 50m means you swim
  50 meters five times on
  only 5 breaths . . .

WEDNESDAY

Running

4-mile timed run

Week # 12

THURSDAY

Swim/PT

10 sets of:
    100m freestyle sprint
    20 pushups
    20 abs of choice

Upper Body PT

Pull-ups: 5 x 2,4,6,8,10
    Regular grip
    Reverse grip
    Close grip
    Wide grip

Arm Haulers: 2 x 75

FRIDAY

Running

3-mile timed run

SATURDAY

Swimming

Hypoxic swim
    5 x 50m,
    50 sec. interval
    4 x 50m,
    55 sec. interval
    3 x 50m,
    1 min. interval
    2 x 50m,
    1 min. interval
    1 x 50m

DO NOT SWIM ALONE!

IF YOU ARE
A BEGINNER

This workout is not specifically designed for people who are out of shape. However, you can alter some of the workouts to build a foundation in order to move on to the more challenging 12-week workout. First, you can test your level of fitness by taking the SEAL PFT.

500 yard swim—If you score above 13 minutes or do not complete:

1. Check your technique by reading Chapter 6 on swimming.
2. Build cardiovascular strength by running, biking or hypoxic swimming (see Week #2 of the 12-week workout, Thursday).

1.5 mile run—If you score above 13 minutes or do not complete:

1. Check your technique by reading Chapter 5 on running.
2. Do the 3-mile Track Workout (see Week #2 of the 12-week workout, Thursday), except change the words "sprint / jog" to "run / walk."

Pull-ups—If you do less than 3 pull-ups:

1. Do **negatives** to build upper body strength. A negative is half of a complete repetition. Simply put your chin above the pull-up bar by stepping up to the bar. Then, slowly let yourself down to the starting position counting to 5. By fighting gravity on the downward motion of the pull-up you are getting your muscles used to lifting your body weight. Eventually, you will be able lift yourself over the bar.

Pushups—If you do less than 30 pushups in 2 minutes:

1. Do negatives until you can do a full pushup.
2. Do pushups on your knees.

Situps—If you do less than 30 situps in 2 minutes:

1. Do crunches, especially if you have lower back problems.

If you still cannot pass the minimum physical standards on the Navy SEAL PFT, you will need to start with the four-week Pre-Training Workout. This is a four-week program that will help you build a foundation of strength and endurance. The workouts may be repetitious, but the best way to build the muscular stamina needed to pass the Navy SEAL PFT is by following these simple steps and finishing the four-week program.

Some general guidelines:

1. Work out five days a week and stretch two times every day.
2. Push yourself until you can no longer perform any of the exercises, and then resort to negative repetitions. Pushing yourself to total muscle failure will quickly increase your scores in pull-ups, pushups, and situps.
3. When running or swimming during the Pre-Training phase, concentrate more on perfecting your technique than on decreasing your times.
4. Stretch for 15 minutes after every workout in order to decrease your pain and soreness the following day.

Follow this workout program and you will be surprised that doing 300 pushups and over 500 crunches in one workout isn't as tough as you thought. After your four-week training program is complete, take the SEAL PFT again and strive to surpass the minimum scores (see page 17).

GOOD LUCK!

Week # 1

MONDAY

Upper Body PT

Regular Pushups 2 x max
   (Do negatives if you
   have to, but stay off
   your knees!)
Wide Pushups 2 x max
Triceps Pushups   2 x max
Regular Pull-ups
   Do a pyramid to your
   max (for example, if
   your max is 5, do
   1,2,3,4,5)
Reverse Pull-ups
   Pyramid down to 1
   from your max
Regular Crunches 2 x 25
Reverse Crunches 2 x 25
Left and Right Crunches 2
   x 50 each side

Max pushups in 1 min.
Max situps in 1 min.
Max pull-ups (no time
   limit)

TUESDAY

Lower Body PT

Squats	2 x 10
Lunges (each leg)	2 x 10
Heel Raises	2 x 10
(each leg)	
Frog Hops	1 x 5

Sprints

20 yd x 5
40 yd x 5
60 yd x 3

Jog 1 mile.
Stretch legs for 15 min.

WEDNESDAY

Running

Jog 1/4 mile
Stretch 10 min.
1.5-mile timed run.
Jog 1/4 mile.
Stretch 15 min.

Week # 1

THURSDAY	FRIDAY	SATURDAY
Swimming	**Run/Swim PT**	REST!
Stretch 10 min. 500 yd sidestroke or breaststroke, timed 500 yd sidestroke technique swim: concentrate on technique! Read Chapter 6 on swimming.	Jog 1/4 mile Stretch 10 min. 1.5-mile timed run 100 yd swim (freestyle) 10 pushups 10 situps Repeat sequence 10 times!	

Week # 2

MONDAY

Upper Body PT

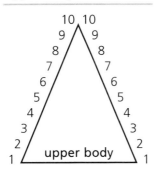

10 10
9 9
8 8
7 7
6 6
5 5
4 4
3 3
2 2
1 upper body 1

Pull-ups x 1
Pushups x 2
Situps x 3
Dips x 2
Each level of the pyramid

Running

Jog 1/4 mile
Stretch for 10 min.
2-mile timed run
Jog 1/4 mile
Stretch for 10 min.

TUESDAY

Lower Body PT

Squats	2 x 15
Lunges (each leg)	2 x 15
Heel Raises	2 x 15
(each leg)	
Frog Hops	1 x 8

Sprints

20 yd x 5
40 yd x 4
60 yd x 3
100 yd x 2

Swimming

500 yds sidestroke
Stretch 10 min.

WEDNESDAY

Running

Jog 1/4 mile
Stretch 10 min.
2-mile timed run
Jog 1/4 mile
Stretch 10 min.

Week # 2

THURSDAY	FRIDAY	SATURDAY

THURSDAY

Same workout as Monday of this week, but swim 500 yds instead of running—give your legs a break!

After you swim:
    Max pushups in 1 min.
    Max situps in 1 min.
    Max pull-ups (no time limit)

FRIDAY

Running

Jog 1/4 mile
Stretch 10 min.
2-mile timed run
Jog 1/4 mile
Stretch 10 min.

SATURDAY

REST!

Week # 3

MONDAY

Upper Body PT

Pull-ups:
   1,2,3,4,5 . . . max, and
      then back down to 1
      (15 sec. break in
      between pull-ups)

10 Super Sets

Regular Pushups	5
Regular Crunches	10
Wide Pushups	5
Reverse Crunches	10
Triceps Pushups	5
1/2 Situps	10

Repeat this sequence 10
   times, for a total of 150
   pushups and 300
   abdominal exercises.
   You have 2 min. to
   complete each set. If
   you finish in 1min. 30
   sec., you have 30 sec.
   rest before the next set.

Running

Jog 1/4 mile
Stretch 10 min.
2-mile timed run
Jog 1/4 mile
Stretch 10 min.

TUESDAY

Running

3-mile timed run

Swimming

800 yd swim

WEDNESDAY

Lower Body PT

Squats	3 x 15
Lunges	3 x 15
Heel Raises	3 x 15
Frog Hops	2 x 8

Sprints

20 yd x 5
40 yd x 4
60 yd x 3
100 yd x 2
220 yd x 1

Week # 3

THURSDAY	FRIDAY	SATURDAY

THURSDAY

Upper Body PT

Pull-ups: 1,2,3,4,5 . . .
   max; then back down
   to 1 (15 sec. break in
   between pull-ups)

15 Super Sets

Regular Pushups	5
Regular Crunches	10
Wide Pushups	5
Reverse Crunches	10
Triceps Pushups	5
1/2 Situps	10

Repeat sequence 15 times,
   for a total of 225
   pushups and 450
   abdominal exercises.

Swimming

500 yd swim

FRIDAY

Running

Jog 1/4 mile
Stretch 10 min.
3-mile timed run
Jog 1/4 mile
Stretch 10 min.

SATURDAY

REST!

Week # 4

MONDAY

Upper Body PT

Pull-ups: 1,2,3,4,5 . . .
max; then back down
to 1 (15 sec. break in
between pull-ups)

15 Super Sets

Regular Pushups	5
Regular Crunches	10
Wide Pushups	5
Reverse Crunches	10
Triceps Pushups	5
1/2 Situps	10

Repeat sequence 15 times,
for a total of 225
pushups and 450
abdominal exercises.

Running

2–3 miles at a comfortable
pace

TUESDAY

Running

Jog 1/4 mile
Stretch 10 min.
3-mile timed run

Swimming

1000 yds sidestroke
Stretch 10 min.

WEDNESDAY

Lower Body PT

Squats	3 x 15
Lunges	3 x 15
Heel Raises	3 x 15
Frog Hops	2 x 8

Sprints

20 yd x 5
40 yd x 4
60 yd x 3
100 yd x 2
220 yd x 1

Week # 4

THURSDAY

Upper Body PT

Pull-ups: 1,2,3,4,5 . . .
    max; then back down
    to 1 (15 sec. break in
    between pull-ups)

20 Super Sets

Regular Pushups	5
Regular Crunches	10
Wide Pushups	5
Reverse Crunches	10
Triceps Pushups	5
1/2 Situps	10

Repeat sequence 20 times,
    for a total of 300
    pushups and 600
    abdominal exercises.

Swimming

500 yds sidestroke

FRIDAY

Running

Jog 1/4 mile
Stretch 10 min.
4-mile timed run
Jog 1/4 mile
Stretch 10 min.

When you have completed
the 4-week training
program, take the SEAL
PFT again. You will be
surprised at how much
your scores will improve.
But don't stop there!

After you achieve the
minimum scores,
I encourage you to keep
training, using the
12-week workout. You
will soon be in the best
physical shape of your life!

NAVY SEAL RECRUITMENT POINTS OF CONTACT

SEAL Detailer
Bureau of Naval Personnel
Pers 401D
Navy Annex
Washington, D. C. 20370
Com. (703) 614-1091
DSN 224-1091

SEAL Recruiter
Naval Special Warfare
2446 Trident Way
San Diego, CA 92155-5494
Com. (619) 437-3641/3656
DSN 577-3641

Officer Detailer
Bureau of Naval Personnel
Pers 415
2 Navy Annex
Washington, D. C. 20370
Com. (703) 614-8327
DSN 224-8327

Dive Motivators (SEAL)
Bldg. 1405
Recruit Training Command
Great Lakes, IL 60088
Com. (708) 688-4643
DSN 792-4643

ABOUT
THE AUTHOR

LT. Stewart G. "Stew" Smith graduated from the United States Naval Academy in 1991. After graduation, he received orders to Basic Underwater Demolition/SEAL (BUD/S) training (Class 182). While on the SEAL teams, he learned to achieve maximum levels of physical fitness thanks to the knowledge of several Chief Petty Officer SEALs, Navy doctors, and nutritionists.

Over half of Stew Smith's life has been devoted to athletics and exercise. From grade school to SEAL training, he has learned and developed several different training regimens. **The Complete Guide to Navy SEAL Fitness** is a reflection of Stew's knowledge and drive to succeed.

After four years on the SEAL Teams, Stew was stationed at the Naval Academy and put in charge of the physical training and selection of future BUD/S students. Since 1995, LT. Stew Smith's use of this workout program has yielded amazing results. The workouts he developed to prepare students for SEAL training are still in use today by SEAL recruiters (The BUD/S Warning Order). And after sending over thirty students to BUD/S, not a single man has quit and all have stated that they were physically prepared.

Stew Smith is also a certified personal trainer and instructor with the Sergeant's Program in the Washington, DC, and Annapolis, MD area.

get FIT NOW.com

The hottest fitness spot on the internet!

Home of:
Five Star Fitness Books and Videos:
ARMY • NAVY • AIR FORCE • MARINES

Featuring
"Ask the Expert" Question and Answer Boards
Stimulating Discussion Groups
Cool Links
Great Photos and Full Motion Videos
Downloads
The Five Star Fitness Team
Insider's Information
Hot Product Reviews
The Navy SEAL Fitness 500
And more!

Log on today to receive a FREE Navy SEAL poster!

Hurry—this is a limited time offer!
While supplies last

www.getfitnow.com

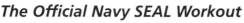